D1710360

THE
GREAT
AMERICAN
FOOD
HOAX

Sidney Margolius

The Great American Food Hoax

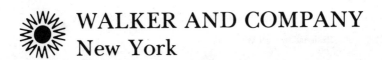

WALKER AND COMPANY
New York

Second Printing—1971

First published in the United States of America in 1971 by the Walker Publishing Company, Inc.

Published simultaneously in Canada by The Ryerson Press, Toronto.

ISBN: 0-8027-0319-4

Library of Congress Catalog Card Number: 72-123269

Designed by Carl Weiss

Printed in the United States of America.

CONTENTS

SECTION I
WHAT'S HAPPENED TO YOUR FOOD?

SECTION II
BUYING THE MOST FOR $100,000

ACKNOWLEDGMENTS

After months of comparing food prices and ingredients for this book, my wife had one terse comment: "It's a jungle."

It is; a jungle of thousands of products, many only slightly different; of manipulative advertising and conflicting claims; varying packages that are hard to compare; temporary specials that try to cloak the general level of high prices but make shopping increasingly complicated.

For helping me find my way through this jungle in order to show you what's behind some of the bushes, I owe special thanks to my wife, Esther, for her unflagging enthusiasm and perceptions; to my research assistant, Mrs. Elaine Jessen, for her astute observations of products and consumers, and for many painstaking surveys and calculations; to David Angevine, former government official and consumer co-op leader, for perceptive analyses of the status of consumer-protection legislation; to Frank Anastasio, executive director of Mid-Eastern Cooperatives, for insights and information over the years; to market-researcher Stefan Josenhans, for his careful surveys of private brands and sale specials; to Dr. W. J. Minor, Chief of Labels, Standards & Packaging Branch of the U.S. Agriculture Department, for generous information, courteously provided; to Dr. Charlotte Schultz for the opportunity to present a consumer view at food conferences sponsored by the Gottlieb Duttweiler Institute in Zurich.

—S.M.

SECTION

I

WHAT'S HAPPENED TO YOUR FOOD?

1

HOW QUALITY HAS GONE DOWN WHILE PRICES HAVE GONE UP

People have been shocked in the late 1960's and early 70's by such prices as 80 cents a dozen for eggs, $1.69 a pound for round steak, even $1.09 a pound for stew beef and $1.39 a pound for pork chops. In many cities milk is now 30 to 35 cents a quart, and American cheese, that traditional low-price staple of moderate-income families, $1 a pound.

This is just the tip of the iceberg. The kind of food you buy has changed too, and at high cost. The public has been gulled into paying some of the most ridiculous prices you ever saw for the ingredients in widely bought ready-to-eat and processed foods.

What has really happened to your food is that you are spending more but eating more poorly. You may not realize you are eating more poorly, but you are.

Even as prices have risen and manufacturers have persuaded the public to pay as much as $3 a pound for 37 cents worth of dried noodles by adding packets of sauce, the nutritional quality of processed foods has deteriorated. This is attributable to the addition of cheap fillers to many processed foods. Curiously, as the cholesterol-worried American public tries to avoid fats for cosmetic and health reasons, the food manufacturers keep feeding them more fats through the unnoticed amounts they now add to hundreds of foods.

This is the age of the adulterated food, the psychologically manipulating package and the skillfully hypnotic supermarket. It is the age of the invented food under an invented name, when a pudding with a vegetable-oil base becomes a "Cool'n Creamy"; a laboratory-concocted powder of sugar, flavorings, vegetable oil and synthetic vitamins becomes the morning's "Start"; a chuck steak becomes a "patio steak"; an "all-meat" frankfurter is 50 percent fat, water, cornstarch and other fillers; and U. S. Grade A frozen broilers have so much water, Europeans are reluctant to buy them in the export market.

To a public already startled by the many additives in foods, one manufacturer has even figured out how to sell just the additive and not bother with the food, in the beverage powder described in Chapter 7, thus demonstrating that housewives today are no longer able to cope with modern food technology. They often simply no longer know what they are buying.

It also is the age when manufacturers pay 5 cents for the package for a breakfast cereal and 4 cents to the farmer for the ingredients, when puzzled and angry housewives actually picket stores and farmers are not sure whom to hate most.

Food now is a $110 billion industry. Its inexorable growth has been fueled by the forced draft of a constant flow of manufactured products.

Because there are these billions at stake, many other things have happened. The food manufacturers are a new political power with as much, if not more, weight than the old farm lobbies. The manufacturers have become a noticeable influence over federal and state agriculture departments and often have effectively stalled moves to defend nutritional quality by such agencies as the Food and Drug Administration, and even by Congress.

The manufacturers also have come to dominate the retailers and many communications media through the power of pervasive advertising that now totals an industry-wide $3 billion a year. Two of the top four advertisers now are grocery manufacturers—Procter & Gamble and General Foods.

The result of this outpouring of products is that supermarkets have gotten bigger and more costly to operate. In just one medium-sized supermarket we counted 151 different types, brands and sizes of breakfast cereals; 63 different brands, types and sizes of tuna and other canned fish; 27 brands and sizes of toothpaste; 48 sizes and types of potato chips, corn chips and similar snacks. In dry cereals alone this supermarket had fifty different kinds in seventeen sizes at eighty-two different prices.

Even if you never buy a sugar-coated crunchy, you pay for such heedless manufacturing and selling practices in the higher prices of the foods you do buy. Supermarket operating costs have gone up from a typical 16 cents of your shopping dollar before World War II to a typical 23 cents today.

Supermarkets' net profits are not the real problem. Their profits are a penny to a penny and a half per dollar, as they always point out in their own defense.

Not even their return on invested capital is the problem, although some consumer spokesmen tend to argue this point when they find themselves stumped by the retailers' penny-a-dollar profit defense.

It is the money that modern supermarkets waste to earn this penny a dollar that has helped to cause this problem. Another cause is the frequent lack of real price competition.

Supermarkets nowadays avoid price competition to a large extent, relying on the semblance of competition through a few specials, but actually competing more strenuously for preferred locations, as in new shopping centers, for attractiveness of interiors and for added services and trading stamps, although this most visible waste is finally beginning to wither in the glare of consumer resentment.

As food manufacturers have become larger, they too have become less competitive on prices, and have concentrated more on nonprice competition such as increased brand-name advertising and slight differentiations in basic products. One, for example, adds a bit of honey to its presweetened cereal; one adds dehydrated vegetables and beef fat to its beef-flavored rice; another adds vermicelli. They often also avoid price competition through different package sizes—one an 8-ounce package, another a 6.

The supermarkets go along. The processed foods such as frozen dinners and vegetables have a higher profit, both in dollars and percentage margins, than do ordinary groceries.

The "marketing spread" itself, which is the cost of bringing foods from the farm to your shopping cart, has risen in our generation from 50 cents of the dollar you pay to 60-62 cents. The farmer now gets an average of only 38-40 cents of that dollar.

In recent administrations, the Agriculture Department itself has become the chief apologist for high prices. While housewives have hit the bricks (a labor term for picketing), and complaints have poured in to Congressmen, the Agriculture Department defends high food prices. It constantly stresses the built-in maid services and great variety at your command (such as the fifty different kinds of dry cereals) and the fact that incomes have risen more than food prices.

In effect, the USDA has become the Pentagon of the food industry. The USDA, for example, tells the public: "New foods often feature 'built-in chef service' as well as 'built-in maid service.' Some are better than those the busy housewife has time to prepare."[1]

At least some may taste better. The food-corporation technologists have become masters of the art of flavoring. But it is hard to understand how an ounce of chicken in a frozen pot pie is "better" for a child, say, than several ounces in a homemade recipe.

The other smokescreen is that "food is a bargain," that it now takes only 17 percent of income. But the "percentage of income" figure used by the Agriculture Department is for the entire public, including institutions, small families, rural families who produce some of their own food, rich families and so on. The U.S. Bureau of Labor Statistics estimates that food takes 22-23 percent of a representative urban wage-earner family's income.

I have long pointed out that the fact that the lower percentage of national income spent on food has nothing to do with the price of food, but is due to higher incomes, arising from a high degree of trade union organization, and because one-third of all wives now work and many husbands have a second job. You too can reduce the *percentage* of your income spent for food by sending your wife out to work or getting a second job, thereby raising your income. But your food still would not be a bargain.

Actually, you are probably paying more for food than even the increase shown in the cost-of-living index, because—if you are at all typical—you now buy more processed foods. Food *expenditures* have been rising faster than food *prices*.

Another claim constantly heard from both the grocery industry and Agriculture Department officials is that food has gone up less than "other items." The fact is that food has gone up more than almost any other *commodity* you buy over the counter. When government officials say food has gone up less than "other items," they are referring to the overall cost of living, including services such as medical care, property taxes and repairs. These have risen especially sharply because they are not amenable to cost reduction through automation. But when you compare food with other commodities (not services), the price of food for use at home went up 22 percent between 1957-59 and 1969 while commodities other than food rose 18 percent, as the USDA Office of Information itself observed with refreshing honesty.

With farmers angry, and threatening almost every year to withhold milk, livestock and other foods from the market, who do you suppose the USDA has been blaming for the problem? Not the middlemen and processors. They are a privileged sanctuary who are praised for their "efficient system of food distribution." The government actually has taken to blaming the consumers. In 1968, then Agriculture Secretary Orville Freeman said, "For many years the farmer has in effect been subsidizing the consumer with low-cost food."

The real beneficiaries of low farm prices have been the manufacturers and distributors. They are the ones the farmer has been subsidizing.

Unfortunately, many extension home economists, agriculture college professors and farm leaders quote the USDA "statistics" and slogans without further investigation. In 1970, the president of Farmland Industries, Inc., a Missouri farmers' cooperative, published ads purportedly defending farmers in the controversy over food prices. The ads argued:

—Other costs are up more than food: services 43 percent, transportation 24 percent and medical care 54 percent.

—Ten years ago it took 21 cents of the take-home dollar to buy food. Last year this was 17 cents.[2]

Sometimes the farmers, or their officials, can't seem to tell their friends from their foes. In late 1970, when pork production was increasing, the National Pork Producers Council advertised to retailers that pork "at normal mark-up is the highest net profit major tonnage item in your meat counter. . . . Stick to your normal mark-up. Prices will be attractive this fall without price cutting."

Actually government policies can raise your food costs despite anything you do to protect yourself. While the Administration was trying to dampen inflation by slowing production and creating unemployment, its Agriculture Department functioned to boost food prices through restraining production, not only through the long-term crop-limiting programs described in Chapter 6, but also of other foods from time to time.

For example, in the spring of 1970, when food costs were at record highs and eggs again had become one of the few reasonably priced protein foods, the USDA warned farmers to reduce their egg-laying flocks to keep up prices. After reaching close to $1 a dozen the previous winter, mainly because of speculation by middlemen, egg prices had fallen about 40 percent as production increased. But at the time the USDA urged production cuts, egg prices still were 3 to 4 cents higher than the previous year.

Similarly, in the spring of 1969 the Agriculture Department issued a regulation limiting supplies of fresh tomatoes coming on the market to larger sizes. In little more than a week prices jumped 5 to 20 cents a pound.

In 1970, farmers acted on their own to force up potato prices by withholding potatoes from the market and even burning some. The farmers' resentment was understandable, although the effect on retail prices during an already rough inflation was harmful. Farmers at that time were getting less than 2 cents a pound for their potatoes, while you were paying 9 to 17 cents.

In fact, the farmers have been getting relatively little benefit from higher retail food prices anyway, and crop-reduction tactics are as futile as the government's anti-inflation efforts. In 1969 the average city family paid $1,173 for farm-originated foods, an increase of $55 or almost 8 percent over the year before. But farmers got only $477 of that expenditure, or $12 more.

Furthermore, even when farm prices go down, retail prices continue their inexorable upward march. From August, 1969, to August, 1970, the farmer's share of the market basket of a year's food actually dropped $3, but the retail cost jumped another $40. By then the middlemen were taking $761 (62 percent) of the $1,237 the city family paid for that market basket.

Sometimes, on such volatile products as bacon, retail price hikes are twice as high as wholesale increases.

The futility of the government's mock war against inflation is that it fails to attack the real cost problems. It is often said that the price of steel affects all other prices. The truth is the other way around. The cost of food represents 25 percent of the labor cost of making steel, cars, houses and all other needs.

Food prices are the real sacred cow, so to speak. Even Congress, while willing to consider minor proposals related to food, has been afraid to come to grips with the gut issue of prices. Congress completely ignored the recommendations of the National Commission on Food Marketing in 1966 for quality grades and other reasonable proposals, even though Congress itself had established the commission to seek ways to restrain food prices.

In 1970 the House Committee on Government Operations similarly refused to take any action on its own subcommittee's report aimed at curbing high meat prices. Because of many complaints, including housewives' boycotts, the special subcommittee had explored ways to hold down prices. But the cattle industry and farm organizations heard about the pending report, and lobbied it to sudden death. The full committee voted for "further study"; in effect, killing the price-curbing effort. It did not even make the report public. The power of the farm organizations was illustrated when a Missouri congressman showed a telegram from the Farm Bureau to explain why he was voting against the report, although his district has large industries with many working families.

The recommendations were mild enough. The subcommittee found:

1. The price increase in the second quarter of 1969 really was excessive. Average retail prices of beef jumped from 89.9 cents a pound in March to 92.7 cents in April, 94.8 cents in May and $1

in June. This sharp increase, unexpected even by the USDA, occurred even though production fell off only 2½ percent. In previous years similar fluctuations in supplies resulted in much smaller price changes.

2. Because of the short supplies and excessive price increases, the subcommittee recommended lifting restrictions on meat imports, mainly boneless lean beef used for hamburger, frankfurters and other processed meats. Lean beef for processing is in especially short supply in our country because of the decline in production of bull and cow beef. Cow meat used for hamburger has become almost as expensive as the grain-fed beef used for steaks and roasts, witnesses at subcommittee hearings pointed out. That is why the price you pay for hamburger has been unusually high in recent years and resistant to declines even when other beef prices do go down a little.

3. The subcommittee also found that the livestock industry plans to restrain future production. The planned increase of only 3 percent a year in beef supplies obviously is inadequate to keep up with increasing demand. The projected increase is even less than the average increase in beef supplies of 4.2 percent a year from 1959 to 1969.

Thus, in the years ahead, you are very likely to be squeezed on the one hand by restrained production, and on the other by higher prices.

The subcommittee felt that the planning for meat supplies cannot be left to the livestock industry alone. For one reason, there has been a big increase since 1965 in large feedlots and a decline in smaller ones. This means a monopoly situation can develop, with even more restrictions on supplies. At congressional hearings in 1969, a representative of a cattle raisers' association said frankly that the association was trying to keep prices up by recommending to its members that they keep production down.

To help solve the supply dilemma, the subcommittee, headed by John S. Monagan of Connecticut, proposed a national commission to gather information on meat requirements.

The recommendation to allow more beef for processing into the country is a sensitive one, feared and resisted by livestock raisers, for understandable reasons. But importing more beef of this type would not affect fed-beef prices seriously, or hurt U.S. livestock growers and packers. It would be in the nature of a temporary device, used from time to time to help keep down price tags on the processed meats on which moderate-income families, especially, depend.

All this is not to say that the government does not provide many useful services for consumers. While USDA consumer services are much less extensive than they were twenty-five years ago, there still are many USDA employees sincerely concerned with consumer needs.

But it is to say that the evidence is that the USDA and even agencies with a prime consumer obligation such as the Food and Drug Administration, often seem more worried about businessmen's reactions than those of consumers. While investigating standards problems for this book, David Angevine was told by an FDA official that the agency was considering revising its standards for fruit drinks and ades to require that labels state the actual amount of real juice (now very little, as shown in Chapter 7). "We are in touch with the industry on this," the official said. Angevine asked if the agency was also in touch with consumers. The official said no, they would not be the ones regulated.

Never underestimate the clout of the food-industry lobby, whether a Republican or Democratic administration is in power. When President Nixon took office, Bryce Harlow, the Washington lobbyist for Procter & Gamble, joined the White House staff. There was an even trade. Mike Manatos, administrative assistant to both President Johnson and President Kennedy, joined Procter & Gamble's Washington office.

With all the problems consumers already have between the government's tin ear, manipulation of foods by manufacturers and juggling of prices by retailers, many who can least afford it themselves waste precious dollars in buying food, observes Frank Anastasio, executive director of Mid-Eastern Cooperatives (a supply organization owned by co-op stores).

Anastasio is especially concerned that items such as canned

sodas and fruit-flavored drinks have their biggest sale in low-income areas. In fact, some of the buying clubs, organized to help low-income families save on food as part of the "war" on poverty, are heavy buyers of canned soda. At least it can be said that by buying wholesale they pay less for nothing.

One problem is that moderate-income families are greatly influenced by TV advertising. Anastasio reports that even the co-ops, while they tried to resist, finally had to stock the flavored sipping straws that were in demand for a while. This product merely added a little flavor to a drink as the child sipped through the straw. As long as the flavored straws were advertised on TV, they sold like mad. As soon as the ads were discontinued, people stopped buying.

Manufacturers increasingly manipulate the public's taste, Anastasio points out. They use cheaper coffee, such as African beans in instant coffee, and now make mayonnaise without egg yolk. The public comes to accept these versions as the standard product. Sometimes, as in coffee, this does not matter nutritionally. But in the case of mayonnaise and peanut butter, which now often has added cooking fat for "smoothness," the nutritional value is affected.

The gradual reduction in the maple syrup content of pancake syrups is another example of the manipulation of taste. Anastasio reports that in 1968 the two leading brands reduced their maple sugar content to 10½ and 11 percent from the previous 15 percent, at the same time raising their prices, not lowering them proportionately or at least maintaining them. The co-op stores kept the maple content of their own-brand syrup at 15 percent even though their supplier had suggested a reduction to 11 percent. In 1970, when we checked this item again, the leading brand (Log Cabin) was down to 6 percent maple sugar, 71.2 percent cane sugar syrup and 22.6 percent corn syrup. Even a leading private brand at a lower price, A&P's Ann Page, had more maple syrup—7.5 percent maple sugar, 2.5 percent honey, and the rest cane and corn syrup. As in other reductions of traditional ingredients, the loss is concealed from your taste buds and eyes by artificial flavorings and caramel coloring.

The increasing proportion of family food money spent on high-priced snacks instead of more nutritious food at less cost is another benefit conferred upon America by the modern food industry. As one of many examples, consumption of potato chips increased 83 percent, and that of carbonated beverages 70 percent during the 1960's. In that period consumption of milk declined.

Total spending for potato chips, corn chips, pretzels and other snack foods is now over $2 billion a year. In 1968 alone, 117 new snack products appeared, the New York State Extension Service reports. Because the bags look big, families don't reckon the costs. They range from $1 a pound for corn chips to over $2 a pound for popcorn.

As another example of the influence of supermarkets, market researcher Stefan Josenhans, in a study of the beer industry, found sales had increased 32 percent from 1958 to 1968, with about 84 percent of beer now packaged and sold by food stores. Altogether (or singly) Americans now guzzle 38 billion 12-ounce cans or bottles of beer a year, at a total expenditure of $6.5 billion.

The general effect of the increased consumption of snack foods and the nutritional cheapening of many processed foods is clear enough. Even while incomes are at record levels and supermarkets stock the boasted abundance of 8,000 different items, the nutritional quality of American diets actually declined from 1955 to 1965.

To the delight of vitamin-pill manufacturers and the obvious dismay of then Secretary Freeman, who for eight years had announced almost every week that food is a bargain, the decline was revealed in a USDA survey made public in 1968. It found:

—Only 50 percent of the families surveyed in 1965 had "good" diets, 20 percent had poor diets and the other 30 percent rated fair.

—The number of "good" diets had declined since the 60 percent figure of the 1955 survey. At the same time, the percentage of families with actually "poor" diets had increased—from 15 percent ten years ago to 20 percent now.

—Money is not the only reason for this decline, since even among families with incomes over $10,000, only 63 percent had good diets. But only 37 percent of families with incomes under $3,000, and only 43 percent with incomes between $3,000 and $5,000 had good diets.

Even the influence of money by itself does not explain why

families are eating more poorly nowadays, when they do have more income than they did ten years ago.

Besides the heavy spending on snacks, families also now are spending a higher percentage of their money on meat, including the reduced-nutrition lunch meats discussed in Chapter 9, and less on such lower-cost sources of protein and other important nutrients as eggs, milk and milk products.

The survey found that families were most likely to short-change themselves in foods containing vitamins A and C, and in calcium. The study especially found that families have cut back on the use of milk and other dairy products that are primary sources of calcium.

The Agriculture Department proposed as one solution to this dangerous trend, more "nutrition education."

"Education" is always a good idea, invariably proposed when a consumer problem is revealed. But it is hardly likely to succeed by itself in the face of the widespread counter-education of TV and promotions of low-nutrition "convenience" foods.

At the 1969 White House Conference on Food, Nutrition and Health, food-industry representatives showed willingness to accept "nutritional" education as a solution to nutritional problems, or, for low-income problems, food stamps, which are as good as cash to them.

What they do balk at are suggestions that food costs be reduced, and that more information about ingredients be put on packages. When I made these proposals to the panel on traditional foods, its chairman, W.B. Murphy, ruled me out of order. He also is the chairman of the Campbell Soup Co.

In fact, many of the panel chairmen and members were officials of large food companies, such as General Foods and McCormick Co., some of whom had battled such potentially useful proposals as the original Truth-in-Packaging law (see Chapter 11).

Apparently, you are going to have to protect yourself as best you can in the supermarkets.

2

HOW YOU CAN PAY TEN TIMES MORE FOR ORDINARY FOODS

Out of the laboratories of America's big food corporations have come many exciting new ways to throw away your money.

The manufacturers have discovered they can dress up ordinary foods with flavorings and inexpensive added ingredients, and charge two to ten times more. Their whole drive now is to turn staples into manufactured products. What was once a distributing industry has become an enormous manufacturing industry—a "growth" industry and a Wall Street favorite.

As you will learn in later chapters, the "convenience food" hoax, with its higher prices and added fillers, has affected many of the foods you buy: frozen vegetables, breakfast cereals, frozen and canned ready-to-eat foods, fruit beverages, low-calorie milks, poultry, meat, cheese and even such staples as bread, rice and noodles.

At a 1968 conference at the Duttweiler Institute in Zurich at which I presented a consumer view to the anger of the manufacturers there, I realized from their statements why these new products carry exaggerated prices. About half of them fail to capture a market even after introduction. Consumers pay for the failures in the prices of the accepted products.

The flood of new food products is rising. The chairman of General Foods, C.W. Cook, revealed in 1970 that this largest food corporation is continuing its new-product development "at a record level." Forced product development is profitable. General Foods reported a 10 percent profit increase, thus qualifying with Wall Street for another year as a growth company.

One of the most revealing examples is the exaggerated prices for new rice and noodle products sold under exotic names and with a few inexpensive additional ingredients or sometimes just flavorings.

Some of these packages can fool you. The manufacturers take a great deal of liberty with the names of the products. Beef Stroganoff with Noodles, for example, is really much more noodles than beef. The pictures of such products show good-sized chunks of beef, chicken and so on, not the little chunks or flakes you really get, if any meat at all.

The packages of Lipton's "one-pot main dishes" look big, with their sloping sides. But all they have inside is a packet of 3 ounces of noodles, a smaller packet of dried sauce ("with lots of tender chicken," the envelope says) and a tiny packet of garnish.

Also, peculiarly, the box lists the cooked serving weight of, for example, 23 ounces. This is after adding 2¼ cups of water. The actual net weight of the contents is usually 5½ or 6¼ ounces, depending on the product.

The true cost also is unusual. We cooked up some of these packages and carefully extracted the lean meat. The Beef Stroganoff, which sells for 79 cents, yielded about 3 ounces of beef, which, with the other minor ingredients, is worth about 30 cents. This means you pay 49 cents for approximately 3 ounces of dried noodles, or at the rate of $2.61 a pound. Ordinary dried noodles cost 37 cents a pound.

The Chicken Baronet yielded about 4 ounces of cooked chicken. That is what they mean by "lots of chicken" for "two adult-size" servings. This much chicken, and the other minor ingredients of the "chicken" sauce such as soy protein, starch, nonfat dry milk and salt, are worth about 23 cents. So you pay approximately 56 cents for 3 ounces of noodles, or at a rate of $2.99 a pound.

The other manufacturers of new rice and noodle products don't charge quite as much—only about two to three times as much as you would pay if you bought the rice or noodles under their own name. Betty Crocker makes it hardest to figure out what you pay. She charges 49 cents for 5.75 ounces of noodles with a prepared dried sauce called Noodles Romanoff. This involves just a little simple arithmetic, which took us about 15 minutes, to figure that it came to $1.36 a pound. Even then you have to add butter and milk, and still cook this product like ordinary noodles.

Or take the inventive Miss Crocker's packaged Macaroni and Cheddar for 49 cents the half-pound box. Since ordinary macaroni costs 31 cents a pound, Betty is really giving us 12 cents worth of dried macaroni and 10 cents worth of cheddar cheese for our 49 cents.

The new flavored rices also can cost you a lot of extra money just for flavorings. Uncle Ben's Beef Flavour'd Rice really costs $1 a pound if you figure it out, compared with 40 cents for his plain converted rice. That "beef flavour" is nothing but beef fat, salt, monosodium glutamate and beef extract. That Uncle Ben looks very kindly in his picture, but he certainly can charge you for his flavoring recipe.

Sometimes you may pay more for the seasoning in modern packaged products than for the basic food. The New York State Extension Service pointed out that such products as Spanish Rice Mix consist of converted long-grain rice with a packet of dehydrated vegetables and seasonings. Six ounces costs 37 cents. A comparable amount of converted long-grain rice costs 12 cents. You pay 25 cents for the seasoning packet.

The actual truth is, you now can pay anywhere from 48 cents a pound for quick-cooking rice to as much as $1.40, depending on what form you buy. Plain instant rice costs 48 cents a pound. But frozen Buttered Rice in a boilable pouch, which sells for 35 cents for a 12-ounce already cooked package, costs you $1.40 in terms of uncooked rice. The so-called butter sauce is really part cornstarch.

One of the most exhorbitant charges is for Mee Tu Fried Rice. This is really ordinary rice, requiring twelve minutes of cooking, plus dehydrated onions, other flavorings and caramel coloring, no less. It is not at all a ready-to-eat fried rice. Ordinary rice would cost you about 5 cents for the 4¾ ounces in the package of seasoned "fried rice" for 39 cents.

Often the convenience itself is illusory. Note that you cook this product as any other quick-cooking rice and then if you want to, the instructions advise, you can fry it. With frozen Buttered Rice, too, you have to cook it for sixteen minutes, compared with five minutes of mere steaming for plain instant rice.

The Food and Drug Administration even has had to act officially to dampen some of the fanciful names, as in the case of Noodle-Roni's Chick'n Almonds. The picture on the package showed a plate heaped with noodles along with a piece of chicken. This, the FDA felt, would indicate that the ingredients in the package would produce a noodle and chicken dinner. But the product contained little or no chicken meat, the agency found; just a packet of sauce mix with unidentified ingredients and a packet of sliced almonds.

The packers of these flavored grain and rice products now more carefully stipulate that they are just flavored. Rice A Roni costs 37 cents for an 8-ounce package of rice-vermicelli mixture with "BEEF Flavour." The word "BEEF" is big and the word "Flavour" smaller. The "flavour" actually more salt than beef extract.

If you are really mad for flavoring, you can add a beef or chicken bouillon cube to ordinary rice, at a cost of a penny per cup of rice, as the New York Extension Service suggests.

Another heavily advertised convenience food devised by food technologists so you can have more time to worry about your budget is Shake'n Bake. It is a striking example of how manufacturers take ingredients that cost pennies a pound and mix, flavor and rename them into "products" that sell literally for dollars a pound. Ordinary bread or soda crackers have a retail value of 25-35 cents a pound. Ordinary flour costs 12 cents a pound. The bread made into toasted crumbs with added flavorings costs 40-60 cents a pound, depending on the brand you buy. Or buy the crackers as cracker meal and the price is 56 cents.

But General Foods is a highly advanced corporation, and has taken the flour and bread crumbs, blended them with a little Crisco and seasonings and brought you Shake'n Bake in packages of 2 3/8 ounces for 27 cents. (The box looks a lot bigger than the packet inside.) This comes to a mere $1.82 a pound, as you can see at once if you can divide fractions in your head. You pay five times as much per pound for the coating as for the chicken.

Shake'n Bake makes Nabisco Cracker Meal look cheap at 33 cents for 9 ½ ounces.

(Note the fractional ounces on these products? The so-called Truth-in-Packaging law was supposed to coax manufacturers to eliminate them. But they are already creeping back.)

The rise in the price of even plain cracker meal itself is a revealing lesson in how a manufacturer big in a particular product line can boost prices out of all proportion to the cost of ingredients or the general rise in food prices. In 1968, cracker meal was 26 cents for the 9 ½ -ounce box (average national price), while flour was 12 cents a pound and bread, 22 ½ cents a pound. By 1970 cracker meal was 33 cents, while flour was still 12 cents and bread, 25 cents. (Nor is prepared cracker meal at 56 cents a pound "a thrifty extender for meat, poultry and fish mixtures," as Nabisco advertises. It costs almost as much as the hamburger and croquettes it is supposed to extend. Oatmeal is both a thriftier and more nutritious extender. So are nonfat milk powder and leftover bread.)

Another fast-selling product from the friendly chemists at General Foods is Cool'n Creamy ready-made pudding. At 45 cents for four half-cup servings, a total of 17 ½ ounces, it is cool'n creamy'n costly. What is it? Certainly it's not much milk, if you think that is what the word "creamy" implies. The ingredients listed, in order of importance, are water, sugar, vegetable oil, nonfat dry milk, starch, thickeners, preservatives, flavorings and artificial color. In eighteen months General Foods spent a cool 5.4 million dollars to promote Cool 'n' Creamy, Philip Dougherty, *New York Times* advertising reporter noted.

The canned puddings are even more expensive—Hunt Snack Pack (15 cents a serving) a little less so than My-T-Fine Rich'n Ready (17 cents).

In comparison, you could make your own puddings from dry mixes for 6 to 8 cents a serving, including the milk you add.

While the Truth-in-Packaging law now requires food processors to say on the package what they mean by a "serving," such as "four half-cup servings," apparently they use different-sized cups. General Foods believes 17½ ounces is four half-cups. The canned puddings provide 20 ounces for four half-cups. The dry pudding mixes also vary in the amount provided for four half-cups.

In 1970 General Foods sent a handsome booklet to editors called *Commitment: A Report on GF's Actions in the Field of Social Responsibility*. Among the examples: how G.F. is providing extra servicing for Kool-Aid soft drink mixes and Good Seasons barbecue sauces for supermarkets in black communities; and how the company is helping to combat pollution, aiding in nutritional education and making "positive responses" to "consumerism."

"Everybody realizes that the old ground rules—the business of business is to make money—no longer apply," says the public relations department's letter to editors.

We are glad to help with G.F.'s new social objectives and diminished enthusiasm for money by pointing out that (1) the plastic bag provided with each small box of G.F.'s Shake'n Bake really adds to pollution; (2) people can buy much more nutrition for their money from foods other than G.F.'s Shake'n Bake and Cool'n Creamy, and (3) G.F.'s Kool-Aid has no nutrition at all, except for sugar and a little synthetic vitamin C at high cost for it, as explained further in Chapter 7.

Ironically enough, notes Betsy Wood, home economist with the Berkeley, California, cooperatives, the 1970 award of the Institute of Food Technologists went to General Foods' Cool Whip. This crowning achievement of the food industry was described as a "stable freeze thaw emulsion resembling whipped cream in appearance, utility and texture when eaten."

Fran Lee, the fighting grandmother of radio and TV, publicly challenged General Foods' announced "social commitment" when it also was promoting products such as Instant Replay, a beverage powder which is 90 percent sugar.

Other convenience foods often with small convenience but large prices are proliferating like weeds. A pancake mix that comes with a paper cup shaker costs three times as much as conventional mixes, New York State extension home economists observe. Refrigerated rolls and biscuits sold in tubes cost four times as much as those with a little dried onion and additional oils than for the plain ones, the USDA *Food and Home Notes* pointed out. One of the many new ready-made spaghetti sauces has water as its leading ingredient. The prepared French dressings can be made at home at one-half to one-third the cost in about three minutes, notes cookbook author Ceil Dyer.

Some of the low-calorie salad dressings even have water as their leading ingredient. You can do that too.

Why do people buy the new food products without understanding what they really provide? Some of the women questioned in a Philadelphia survey were seeking economy and convenience. These were mothers of large, middle-income families, and among the products listed, they tended especially to try whipped toppings and orange-flavored breakfast drink powders and concentrates.[3] But their desire for economy obviously exceeded their know-how or the information available to them.

For middle-aged higher-income families, trying new products often reflected a search for fewer calories and convenience but also seemed a kind of status symbol. They tended to report that they usually tried these products before their friends did.

But the natives are getting restless.

An observant woman in Santa Monica sent me the label of a frozen "cook-in-bag" product called Crem'd Style Gravy & Sliced Chicken. Note the spelling of "Crem'd." A luscious "suggested serving" picture showed four slices of turkey and a little gravy on a slice of bread. But the ingredients mentioned no "Crem," whatever that is. The leading ingredient was gravy. Its ingredients were, in order of importance, water, flour, starch, salt and vegetable fat. The package we checked, at 29 cents for 5 ounces, yielded four paper-thin slices of chicken roll of three-inch diameter, totaling a little over 1 ounce, and 4 ounces of gravy. The reason the serving looked generous in the picture is that it was shown on a relatively small plate, like the joke about the restaurant that used small waiters to make its portions look big.

This woman was amused at what she said was truly a mouthful of chicken. Another woman was fighting mad. She wrote: "I bought a package of frozen Gravy & Sliced Turkey, weight two pounds, for $1.49. When this was baked there were about four cups of gravy and not enough turkey to serve one person, and there were four of us. For 75 cents a pound, I would expect a fairly good serving of meat."

There is more to tell about this product later. But first, consider another woman's beef. She sent it to me through the mail. It was a sample of luncheon meat, which arrived smelling very strong. (I would urge readers of this book to send such samples to the manufacturers or supermarkets instead of to me.) She wrote: "When I pay a dollar for food I expect my dollar's worth. We use lunch meat a couple of times a week because I have a son in school and my husband takes lunches. Most of the time lunch meat is loaded with fat, and its contents are strong tasting. Most families buy lunch meat. Do they all get beat with plastic wrappers, extra casings, all kinds of fat and pickles and olives to add to the weight?"

The answer, unfortunately, is that many probably do get beat. As explained in Chapter 9, regulations permit up to 30 percent fat and 10 percent water in luncheon meats.

Bill Gold, *Washington Post* columnist, who has a sharp eye for the ridiculous and a friendly ear for consumers, wrote:

This is the panel from a frozen food product. Can you figure what it is?

"Water, corn syrup, shortening, sugar, whey solids, food starch-modified, dextrose, sodium caseinate, flavoring, gelatin, whole milk solids, monosodium and di-glycerides, salt, vinegar, polysorbate No. 60, vanilla, monosodium phosphate, guar gum, lecithin, artificial color, in a crust of wheat flour, sugar, shortening, water, dextrose, graham flour, sorghum grain flour, salt, sodium bicarbonate, ammonium bicarbonate, artificial flavoring and coloring."

Give up? Why it's lemon cream pie, of course. Isn't that the way *you* make it?

What our indignant friends do not understand—along with almost 200,000,000 other Americans—is the subtle labeling and glamorized "suggested servings" permitted by present regulations and the way they are administered. The rules are so subtle that they permit all kinds of foolery and waste.

The way things are, you have to watch the names of foods and the lists of ingredients like a hawk if you want to survive in the food-processing jungle. You even have to carry in your head such distinctions as that a product labeled "mayonnaise" must have 65 percent oil, but "salad dressing" can have only 30 percent.

Under present regulations, as administered by the Food and Drug Administration, and for products containing poultry and meat by the U.S. Agriculture Department, the packer is required to list the ingredients in order of importance if these agencies have not established a "standard of identity" for the product. There are eighteen identity standards established by the FDA, including standards for margarine; mayonnaise, French dressing and salad dressing; canned fruits and juices; jams and jellies; canned vegetables; frozen desserts such as ice cream; cheese and cheese products; macaroni and noodles.

The USDA has established two identity standards, for corned beef hash and chopped ham.

A manufacturer need not list ingredients on a product for which there is an identity standard, if the product meets it. For most of the modern processed foods, especially the proliferating convenience items, there are no identity standards, and the ingredients must be listed.

A wary, highly literate consumer can find the ingredient lists somewhat useful. In the case of the Gravy & Sliced Turkey, the fact that "Gravy" comes first means there is more gravy than turkey. Moreover, if the woman who bought this product had read the list of ingredients in fine print (food labels are getting as bad as insurance policies), she would have seen that under "Gravy," the first item listed is water. This means that water is the leading ingredient in the gravy. The other ingredients, in order of importance, are starch, flour, salt, vegetable fat, chicken fat, turkey giblets, various flavorings and caramel color—an obvious concoction of inexpensive fillers.

Then under "Turkey" the label shows a separate list of ingredients: "turkey, natural juices, salt, brown sugar, sodium phosphates, hydrolyzed vegetable protein, flavoring, sodium erythorbate." While this version of "turkey" might well win the American Chemical Society's annual award for new advances in chemistry, a close reading shows how relatively little turkey there is in the 2-pound package.

But the problem is that both the "standard of identity" and "list of ingredients" rules have been made obsolete to a large extent by the rapid development of ready-prepared foods, and the difficulties of shopping in crowded supermarkets with their multitude of different brands, variations, sizes, etc.

A housewife obviously cannot be expected to memorize all the standards already in existence for corned beef hash, pork and beans, peanut butter and many other foods, let alone the new ones being developed in the literally-panting and sometimes futile race of government agencies to keep up with new products.

As a matter of fact, she would find it almost impossible to learn what the standards are. The Appendix at the end of this book provides what is probably the most complete list of standards for meat, poultry and fish products yet published for the general public. Elsewhere in this book we tell about the standards for a number of other products, including cheeses and bread, and some canned goods.

But to show the difficulty the ordinary consumer encounters in learning what the standards are, Angevine, himself a former government official, commented:

FDA has issued eighteen standards of identity, quality, and container fill. Each standard covers a group of products. They are quite detailed and difficult for the layman to understand. Part 19, Cheese & Cheese Products, takes 54 pages in the *Federal Register;* Part 20, Frozen Desserts, 40 pages; Part 27, Canned Fruits & Juices, 44 pages; Part 51, Canned Vegetables and Vegetable Products, 17 pages; and Part 53, Canned Tomato Products, a blessed five pages.

If I as a consumer wonder how much chokecherries are in the jar labeled "Chokecherry Jelly," I go to the U.S. Courthouse nearest my home, locate the *Federal Register,* browse through the index under "Food," "Jellies," and "Chokecherries," and finally locate Part 29, Fruit Butters, Jellies, Preserves. Here, if I am alert, intelligent, and highly motivated, I find what I'm looking for.

Or, if I know that FDA is responsible for such standards, I can write FDA. Chances are they'll send me Part 29. However, FDA may direct me to the Superintendent of Documents, who has this item on sale for 15 cents.

Also, the standards often are surprisingly low, as you will discover in later chapters on specific products.

What is really needed is a requirement that labels give the

actual amount of at least the main ingredients, whether or not an identity standard has been established. If the label said plainly that the jar labeled "chicken with noodles" has at least 15 percent chicken, and the "noodles with chicken" 9 percent, a shopper would have some factual information on which to decide whether the extra price is worth the extra chicken, or to compare prices among different brands, as well as the different versions.

Some of the terminology used in lists of ingredients also may confuse you, especially the word "moisture," often used on cheese products. This is, of course, simply water.

Similarly, merely listing ingredients in order of importance falls short of today's informational needs. For example, many processed meats such as bologna and franks list water as a second leading ingredient, but do not state the amount. Thus the shopper can never know whether one brand has 10 percent water and another 5 percent.

At present the FDA does not even require that the ingredients lists be shown on the front panel of the package or in reasonably legible type. Usually they are shown on the side or back, often under the latest premium offer, and in quite small type. Ingredients lists on side panels may not be noticed at all when the product is on the shelf or in the freezer cabinet.

The Agriculture Department's policy of letting food manufacturers show pictures of "suggested servings" also has facilitated the fooling of consumers. Many devices are used to glorify the actual portions provided, while remaining within the letter of the regulations.

This is not to criticize all modern processed foods. Some offer a measure of convenience at not too high a cost, or even at a saving, as in frozen orange juice. The flavorings are a tribute to the food technologists. There may come a time when a young husband will complain that his mother's factory cooked better than his bride's. Nor is there any suggestion, nor even any way, that corporations should be forbidden to invent new combinations, except possibly for some of the almost wholly synthetic products.

But the public at least deserves to be told just how much of what is in the product. The need has become increasingly urgent with the development of meat "analogs." These are substitutes for meat manufactured to have much the same taste and appearance. Usually the meat substitutes or meat extenders (used in combination with meat) are made of soybean or other grain or vegetable protein. These substitutes or extenders already are increasingly used in canned and frozen ready-to-eat dishes, in soup mixes and as a substitute for bacon strips or bits, as in those sold under the BacOs and Stripples brand names.

While vegetable proteins are not as complete in amino acids as those from animal sources, some of the analogs have their own advantages in certain cases. For example, Stripples, the new striplike bacon analog, made of a combination of wheat and soy protein, has little or no cholesterol and only one-third the calories of bacon. Market tests showed it to be acceptable to consumers.[4]

But, as Helen Nelson, executive director of the Illinois Consumer Association, has pointed out, if adding soybean extender to hamburger, for example, makes it lower in cost, then the savings should be passed on to the consumer and should not result merely in more profit for the processor. The consumer has a right to know whether he is getting such extenders, and how much, this forthright consumer spokesman warns.

Because the government agencies are unable to develop identity standards at the rate that new products spill onto the market, and because they tend to set standards on the basis of existing practices even if low, they could accomplish more sooner by requiring that percentages of ingredients be shown, and that the lists be displayed on the front panel in more noticeable type.

At present, many people seem unaware even of the key fact that the list of ingredients is arranged *in order of predominance*, probably since the labels do not point this out.

Even cats get more facts than humans. Pet foods are required to show on their labels the exact amount of "moisture" (water) in the product.

But the chairman of the National Association of Food Chains, Bert Thomas, who also is president of Winn-Dixie Stores in the South, complained that if the demand for lists of nutrients is heeded, "we'll be so busy cluttering up the label with so much information that wouldn't be used it would lose its selling appeal."[5]

Even when a consumer directly asks a manufacturer what the ingredients are, all he is likely to get is doubletalk, as an enterprising student at Geneva College recently learned. Leonard Penczak, a student of Dr. Stewart Lee, economics department chairman, wrote to ten large food and toiletries companies, asking why their products do not list ingredients on the label.

If you translate the responses to Penczak's inquiries, they fall into four types: (1) "We give you all the information you simpletons can understand"; (2) "We don't list our ingredients because we don't have to"; (3) "We don't list for competitive reasons"; (4) "Why not be your own guinea pig?"

For example, Penczak wrote to the Gillette Company, saying he had looked at the can of "new Foamy Surf Shaving Cream" for the ingredients, but found only that it contained Hexachlorophene. A man with an allergy or skin condition might need to know more, Penczak pointed out.

Gillette gave a mystifying "simpleton" type of reply: "It has been our experience that because of the differences in nomenclature for chemicals used by toiletries and cosmetic companies, and also because of the use of trademarks to identify ingredients rather than the proper chemical name, a listing of ingredients could mislead rather than inform. If a consumer with an allergy to one or more identified substances has asked, we have always told him whether any of our products contain such substances. . . ."

The Stanley Home Products Co. gave a be-your-own-guinea pig answer: ". . . a list of chemical names [of] ingredients of our Creme Rinse would not really be helpful. . .comprehensive toxicity tests were performed on Creme Rinse with no adverse results. . . . Of course, this does not mean that a very small number of persons might not be allergic. . . . If your wife is concerned about this, she might first apply a small amount in an inconspicuous part of her scalp to see if she experiences any reaction."

Kraft, in effect, said "We don't have to," in relation to its Miracle Whip: "There [are] 17 foods for each of which a definition and standard of identity has been decided upon by the FDA. . . . If a product in this group conforms to the standard recipe...the maker is not required to identify the ingredients...."

Having refused to give any information, Kraft thereupon invited Penczak to write again if he had any further questions. If he did, you can be sure he would not get any further answers.

The manufacturer of Del Haven grape jam provided an interesting insight into the fact that some processors think eventually they will have to provide more information, even though he declined to give it now: "It is my opinion that in the next few years all foods will have to have an ingredient statement, but for the time being, none is needed on grape jam...."

Of the ten companies, only Best Foods did state the ingredients in their reply, but gave the usual explanation that they did not have to do so on the label because their Hellman's Mayonnaise met the standard.

Some signs of recognition of the need for more informative labeling are appearing among government officials. At the 1969 House Consumer Subcommittee hearings on food labeling, Dr. Robert K. Somers, USDA Deputy Administrator for Consumer Protection, agreed that percentage labeling of ingredients could be useful to consumers, as reported by *U.S. Consumer,* a Washington newsletter.

Under a plan announced by the FDA late in 1970, baby foods and infant formulas would have to show on their labels such information as the quantity of protein, and carry a warning that the product should not be used as the sole source of protein if it falls below specified levels. Nutritional requirements for baby foods are especially important. Some are reported to contain so much starch and water that they yield only 12 percent solid food.

Actually, with the assent and guidance of their pediatricians, mothers often could control the nutritional quality of baby foods more dependably by preparing some baby foods themselves from family food, as well as save 15 to 25 percent of the costs. For one reason, the protein in different commercially prepared baby "dinners" of cereal, meat and vegetables ranges considerably—from 2 to 4 percent by weight and in "high-meat" dinners of meat and vegetables, from 6 to 8 percent (although this information is not always made available to the purchasers).

Too, manufacturers have tended to add seasonings for the sake of the mother who tastes the food to see if it is suitable, rather than for any real need or desire by the baby. After widespread criticisms, manufacturers have eliminated monosodium glutamate which had been widely used in baby foods.

Until recently, at least, they also added salt "far in excess of those that nature gave to vegetables, meats and various mixtures," Dr. Lewis K. Dahl, head of the Research Medical Service at Brookhaven National Laboratory, has pointed out. Dr. Dahl noted that "a baby's needs for salt are amply satisfied by the salt that it gets from either mother's or cow's milk." The danger of overuse of salt is, of course, hypertension (high blood pressure).

Thus, even more than in other ready-to-eat foods, it is important to check the list of ingredients carefully to note the relative prominence of flavorings such as salt, and other additions you or your pediatrician may consider unnecessary or even undesirable.

Pediatricians sometimes prefer brand-name prepared formulas because they have vitamins and minerals added. Too, if the baby is not doing well on one brand the doctor can try another. The various formula manufacturers aim tremendous promotions at the doctors. Still, mothers must be guided by their pediatricians' advice (among other reasons, because of any need for added vitamins such as vitamins C and D or minerals such as iron).

But it is noticeable that the protein in various brands of canned prepared formulas varies considerably and most do not have even the percentage of protein of a home-prepared formula using evaporated milk. Some canned formulas, in fact, have less than half the protein in evaporated-milk formulas even though their ingredients, often vegetable fat and skim milk, are much cheaper. The proposed FDA regulations would require that formulas and other baby foods meet minimum levels of protein, vitamins and minerals or else carry a statement that additional quantities should be supplied.

But beyond baby foods, the FDA also has started an investigation to determine whether minimum and maximum nutrient levels for ready-to-eat and other processed foods should be established. Dr. Jean Mayer, who directed the 1969 White

House Conference on Food, Nutrition and Health pointed out that the nature of our food supply is changing: "It is no longer enough to guarantee the wholesomeness of food. We also now need guidelines for processed foods, which now constitute more than half our food supply."

But a proposal in 1971 by the FDA, with the approval of some manufacturers, for listing nutritional values under scientific names poses a new danger even though these plans have been praised by some half-knowledgeable "consumer advocates." Labeling of foods by content of various vitamins, etc., opens the way to more of the kind of economic hoaxery that already has developed. As with watered fruit drinks, ready-to-eat cereals, etc., manufacturers can add cheap synthetic vitamins and proclaim that some synthetic powder or beverage which is largely water, provides "100 per cent of your vitamin C" needs. For protein, too, manufacturers would (and sometimes already do) add cheaper sources such as soybean derivatives and nonfat milk powder.

Food manufacturers are only too willing to add vitamins or other enrichment to cheap foods and beverages and secure a nutritional blessing. Another example is the new "enriched fish sticks" (merely made with enriched flour). "Nutritional labeling" may well start a wasteful and confusing fortification horsepower race.

If products are labeled with percentages of ingredients under common food names such as beef, peas, sugar, water, added fat, etc., then an additional declaration of nutritional values could be useful, such as a listing by percentages of daily requirements of various nutrients supplied by the product.

CHAPTER

3

THREE BITES OF MEAT: THE REAL PRICE OF READY-TO-EAT DINNERS

Consumers become understandably irate on buying various frozen and canned ready-to-eat dinners and finding very little meat floating in a lot of sauce. One man wrote to me, "Have you opened a can of beef stew lately? It used to contain large chunks of beef, enough for two people. I just opened two cans and all that was in them were three or four bite-sized pieces of meat and all the rest was potatoes, carrots and gravy!"

One determined woman carefully removed the crust from a chicken pot pie, picked out the meat and vegetables from the gravy and reported there was less than an ounce of chicken meat, three tiny carrot slivers, a few peas and what she called "some vegetable debris."

A San Francisco man sent in the label from a combination package of a Chicken Chow Mein dinner which had a total marked weight of 2 pounds, 11 ounces. He underscored the admonition on the label to drain the vegetables and "DISCARD LIQUID." "You throw away one pound of this package," he wrote in amazement. "One pound is water. You have one pound, 11 ounces left."

The proliferation of canned and frozen ready-to-eat foods has made a real shopping puzzle for consumers. Many working wives, small families, harassed mothers and single persons now use these often. The actual portions you get in different types and brands vary. Some are relatively fair buys for the price or can be improved with a few quick additives. Others are ridiculous. In few cases do these heat-and-serve products reach the level of ingredients in standard home recipes for the equivalent cooked dishes.

The amount of actual nutrients you get for your dollar is what you really need to know in order to compare values in such foods. But the consumer has to shop almost blind. As pointed out in Chapter 2, present labeling laws are completely obsolete, since labels merely must list the ingredients in order of importance, not tell the amounts of each.

Nowhere is this lack of information more apparent, often misleading and disappointing, and potentially harmful nutritionally, than in the heat-and-serve dinners.

Let the record show that my wife, Mrs. Elaine Jessen and I separated, extracted, drained and weighed scores of ready-to-eat dinners, pot pies, canned stews and other heat-and-serve dinners and breakfasts.

The results are not encouraging. In most cases, the products we checked measure up to the total net weight and the government standards for the meat ingredients, with some exceptions, such as an eighth of an ounce here and there.

But the government standards themselves are low. Only once in a while did the meat ingredient in heat-and-eat products we checked exceed the minimum standard.

Ready-to-eat dinners can serve a useful purpose at times. Consumers do not, of course, expect them to cost the same as home-prepared meals. Even the actual going prices—frozen dinners tend to cost two to two and a half as much as equivalent home-prepared versions—would not be the main stumbling block (although a significant extra cost for family meals) if the ingredients were less adulterated with fillers such as added starch, sauces, breading and thickeners, and if the main portions were nearer home-prepared versions.

Some of the cheapening of ingredients is ridiculous, as in the breading on fried chicken pieces in a heat-and-serve dinner, which represented 37 percent of the weight of the small pieces of chicken.

Small savings on ingredients can, of course, accumulate into large profits. Another problem is that competition in packaged foods often seems to move toward cheapening rather than improving quality in an era when quality is hidden behind a package or can.

A case in point is the *Wall Street Journal* report on the profit performance of the Jiffy Foods Corp., a frozen foods packager. This company formerly put 40 percent meat and 60 percent gravy in frozen meat dishes. Then it realized that it was selling 1½-pound packages at higher prices than its chief competitor got for 2-pound packages with 25 percent meat and 75 percent gravy. Jiffy adopted its competitor's ratio and reported that its profits rose 329 percent in six months.

A look at the standards for canned and processed meat, poultry and fish products (see Appendix) will show just what you can expect in any of the ready-to-eat foods—which is not very much. For example, a frozen beef dinner must provide at least 25 percent meat figured on the total meal minus any appetizer, bread and dessert. Frozen egg rolls must provide at least 10 percent meat; beans with frankfurters in sauce, at least 20 percent franks; canned beef stew, at least 25 percent meat; ham spread such as deviled ham, at least 50 percent; canned ravioli, at least 10 percent meat in the ravioli; frozen lasagna with meat and sauce, at least 12 percent meat.

As you can see from these samples, the amounts can be small. The ravioli meat content, for example, is exclusive of sauce. A 16-ounce can may have 40 percent or more sauce. This leaves less than 10 ounces of ravioli. Thus, the entire meat content of the 16-ounce can may be less than 1 ounce on an uncooked basis.

The poultry standards are even lower. Chop Suey (American Style) with Macaroni and Meat must contain at least 25 percent raw beef or other meat when cooked. But a product labeled Chicken Chop Suey (or Chow Mein) need have only 4 percent chicken meat (cooked basis). In comparison, a home recipe would have about 30 percent. A heat-and-serve chicken or turkey dinner need have only 18 percent cooked meat; a canned chicken or turkey soup, only 2 percent meat. You can select others for citation yourself.

Questioned about the permitted lower amounts, W.J. Minor, Chief of the USDA Labels, Standards and Packaging Branch, points out that one reason for the lower poultry standards is that the poultry items are computed on a cooked basis, and the beef and other meat items are on an uncooked basis (except where noted otherwise in the Appendix).

But another reason, Dr. Minor explains, is the precedent set by historical preparation practices, especially for the Chinese-style heat-and-serve products. (Apparently the reasoning of the food processors is that if an Oriental can live on a handful of rice, an added ounce of chicken should make an American standard of living.)

Actually, the meat content in ready-to-eat products was even lower before USDA revised its standards during the 1960's after years of complaints from consumers wrangling with the food industry. Borden & Co., manufacturers of Lipton dehydrated soup, even went to the Supreme Court to try to prevent the USDA from requiring that canned or dehydrated poultry soups have at least 2 percent chicken. But the distinguished justices knew what the founding fathers would consider chicken soup, and ruled for 2 percent—not really either a profile in courage or a great advance for consumers. It only took three years to effectuate this requirement.

Before the mild improvements in standards, you got even less of the more-important ingredients—usually only 51-54 percent fish in fish sticks, compared with the present 60 percent minimum (and the usual 67-69 percent in home-prepared versions.)

The main value of the standards is that they keep these low levels of ingredients from sinking even lower. But they are little help to the consumer in shopping or comparing values. To know what you are buying, you would have to memorize an extremely long list.

You also would have to keep in mind such distinctions as that a product labeled Beef with Gravy has at least 50 percent beef, but one labeled Gravy with Beef has only 35 percent; that Chili con Carne with Beans has only 25 percent beef and Chili Sauce with Meat only 6 percent; that Chop Suey (American Style) with Macaroni and Meat has at least 25 percent meat, but Chop Suey Vegetables with Meat only 12 percent; that Spaghetti Sauce and Meat Balls must have at least 35 percent meat balls on a cooked basis, but Spaghetti with Meat Balls and Sauce only 12 percent, and Spaghetti Sauce with Meat, only 6 percent; that Boned Chicken must have at least 90 percent meat, skin and fat, but Boned Chicken with Broth only 80 percent, and a baby food called Chopped Poultry with Broth only 43 percent; that Lightly-Breaded Shrimp must have at least 65 percent shrimp, but Breaded Shrimp only 50 percent.

An important point to note in your own buying is that manufacturers add convenience to convenience. For example, frankfurters are a convenience food and so are canned beans. But when manufacturers put them together in one can, the cost rises disproportionately.

Margolius's law is that as real convenience decreases, the price of the product increases geometrically.

The Heat-and-Serve Meals

Because of their wide use, we made a special investigation of heat-and-serve meals, often also called TV dinners, which more properly is the Swanson brand name.

In general, the price of such meals as frozen turkey and chicken dinners at a typical 65 cents is about twice the estimated cost of 30 to 40 cents for preparing dinners of similar-sized servings at home, even if convenience ingredients such as turkey roll, canned peas and instant mashed potatoes are used. For a family of four the difference in cost would be a significant $1.20.

The costlier Swanson Turkey Dinner (65 cents), labeled 11 ½ ounces, did yield that weight even after heating. It provided 2 ½ ounces of turkey, 2 ounces of peas, 3 tablespoons of stuffing, a small serving of cranberry sauce and gravy.

The less expensive Morton's Turkey Dinner (45 cents) yielded the same amount of turkey and approximately the same amount of vegetables.

All the brands actually yielded a little more turkey meat than the approximately 2.1 ounces called for by the USDA minimum standard.

Both Swanson's and Morton's romanced the buyer with their picture of the serving shown on the package. The Swanson picture showed three rather thick slices of turkey and perhaps a fourth. Actually, there was one thin slice and some very small pieces under that. The Morton's package similarly showed substantial-looking slices. The actual portion consisted of small slices and shreds.

The picture of the franks on Morton's Beans with Franks frozen dinner exaggerated the size of the actual franks by a quarter to half an inch. When such small franks (about 3 ½ inches) are involved, that is a noticeable difference.

Swanson's frozen breakfast used another and rather artistic device. The sausage patties in the picture were actual size, but were shown in a little smaller compartment, so they seemed relatively larger.

Some of the pictorial exaggerations are more ludicrous than a serious economic issue. Swanson's frozen Noodles and Chicken Dinner showed a sprinkling of peas in the picture. There were actually three peas. We have three witnesses to that—one for each pea. Carrots were listed in the ingredients, but were not visible in the dinner. The small bits of chicken look more prominent in the picture, in relation to the reduced size of the tray, than in the actual serving.

USDA regulations require that pictures or "vignettes" accurately represent the enclosed products. In actual practice, often they do not.

What do you get in a Fried Chicken Dinner? We got a small drumstick, thigh and wing, weighing a total of 5 ½ ounces. After removing the breading (2 ounces) and bone, the yield of boned chicken was 2 ½ ounces—again slightly exceeding the minimum standard. We also got 2 ounces of mixed vegetables and 2 ¾ ounces of mashed potatoes. The apple and peach slices emphasized on the package came to 1 ¼ ounces.

The three brands of beef dinners we dissected also met at least the government standard (yielding at least 2 ½ ounces) and one, Sultana (A&P's private brand) actually yielded 3 ½ ounces, no small miracle, since it cost only 38 cents, compared with the 59- to 65-cent prices of the national brands. It also even had a little more solid food and less gravy than the national brands.

The more exotic frozen dinners, such as Veal Parmigiana, "international dinners" such as German and Mexican, Fried Shrimp and so on, all carry higher prices than the standard turkey, beef and fried chicken dinners, but yield the same small portions, especially of the meat or fish component.

The less expensive frozen dinners on the market in the 40-45-cent bracket use such cheaper ingredients as beans and franks, spaghetti and meat balls and noodles. These dinners have little or no advantage in convenience of preparation over the canned versions, and are more expensive even than the overpriced canned combinations discussed later in this chapter. Frozen noodle and chicken dinners, in our experience, often supply only 1 ounce of boned chicken meat.

The noodles and chicken component, deducting the value of the other components, had an estimated cost of 36 cents for 9 ounces, costlier even than the rather expensive (for what you get) Noodles with Chicken in jars.

A Beans with Franks dinner at a seemingly low 39 cents for 12 ounces, in our experience yielded slightly over 1 ½ ounces of franks. We estimated that you could warm up, in less time, an equivalent dinner, using all ready-made ingredients, such as canned beans, for 19 cents.

Frozen spaghetti with meat balls yielded 4 ounces of meat balls and 6 ½ ounces of spaghetti with sauce. The rest is cooked sliced apples and a half slice of bread. That part of the price attributable to the spaghetti and meat balls costs the consumer about 45 percent more than canned spaghetti and meat balls, itself an overpriced product.

A frozen macaroni and cheese dinner costs twice as much as canned macaroni and cheese.

An even more serious concern is the widely sold 2-pound package of frozen Gravy and Sliced Turkey mentioned in Chapter 2. Apparently the fact that the word gravy comes first has not been sufficient to warn consumers, especially since the picture on the big package shows a relatively small bowl of gravy, compared with the pictured platter of turkey.

The gravy in one sample after heating weighed 16 ounces and the sliced turkey not quite 8 ounces, a total of about 24 ounces, although the package weighed the marked 2 pounds (32 ounces) before heating. The second sample after heating yielded 8 ounces of turkey and 19 ounces of gravy, a total of 27 ounces.

If this much loss is attributable to evaporation during heating, and whether or not the gravy contains unnecessary water which results in a large degree of evaporation, what has disappointed buyers who complained to me is that there is little turkey in what looked like a big box for $1.49. The thin slices appear to be turkey roll, available at a cost of $1.25 a pound or about 65 cents for a half a pound. If anyone really wanted that much gravy, canned gravy can be bought at a cost of about 31 cents for two cups.

Similar frozen products are Gravy and Sliced Beef and Gravy and Sliced Chicken. The New York Extension Service found that frozen Salisbury Steak and Gravy at the same prices (65 to 93 cents a pound) provided more meat than Gravy and Beef.

Big 2-pound packages of frozen chow meins on the market at seemingly low prices also yield low amounts of the chicken and shrimp components. In the case of one brand of Chicken Chow Mein, despite the picture of large lumps of chicken, the list of ingredients shows that there is less chicken than celery or onions.

What can you expect in an 8-ounce frozen pot pie? Typically, about 1 ounce of meat (occasionally 1 ¼ ounces), 2 to 2 ½ ounces of crust, about an ounce or less of potatoes, peas or carrots and 2 ½ ounces of broth. The vegetables may consist, as in one sample, of seventeen peas and eight bits of carrot.

Although, at sale prices of under 25 cents, pot pies are a moderate value, a can of condensed poultry or beef soup at a little less cost yields about 50 percent more solid food. Usually the chicken in frozen pot pies is about 40 percent less than that of home-prepared versions, and beef in beef pies is about 27 percent less.

In general, you can estimate that you get 53 cents worth of poultry meat value for the dollar you spend for *canned* whole or boned chicken, but only 17 cents worth when you buy frozen chicken pot pies, 20 cents worth when you buy a frozen chicken dinner and as little as 10 cents worth from some of the other frozen poultry-containing foods.[6]

Similar problems have arisen among the popular frozen fish products. There is no doubt that the ready availability of fish in frozen form all year around at relatively reasonable prices has been a real boon to consumers. But when packers went beyond selling frozen uncooked fish, and developed the many frozen cooked fish items now on the market, the nutritional value deteriorated.

For example, frozen breaded shrimp by law need have only 50 percent shrimp. Frozen fish cakes have only about 60 percent of the protein value of a standard home recipe.

Frozen precooked foods tend to be sold at an administered or cost-plus price, rather than on the basis of market quotations of the main ingredient, such as poultry meat. In fact, several items of the same type may be similarly priced, despite a difference in the cost of their ingredients; for example, turkey, chicken and beef dinners may be priced much the same.

The More Convenient Egg

The frozen omelets introduced in 1970 offer an opportunity to pay 30 cents for 10 cents worth of ingredients. But look at the convenience. You save the work of breaking an egg. But when you cook your frozen ham omelet you may find, as we did, that the picture on the package makes the bits of ham seem disproportionately larger (by reducing the size of the surrounding egg), and that the fourteen bits shown turn out to be three bits of ham and eleven pieces of gristle.

We estimate that a container gives you an egg and a half, worth about 7 cents at late 1970 prices, plus about 3 cents worth of other ingredients.

The Swanson frozen breakfasts provide a little more actual convenience (if you remember to start heating one twenty minutes before you're ready for breakfast), and somewhat more food for the money. In the scrambled egg breakfast you get about 24 cents worth of egg, sausage patty and potatoes for your 47 cents.

Three Forms of Pizza

In a revealing survey in 1969, the New York State Extension Marketing Service compared different forms of pizza, one of the most popular nationality foods. The service noted that three different forms—refrigerated, dry mix and frozen—and sixteen different brands of pizza were included in a recent supermarket survey of nationality foods. Pizza mix involved the most home preparation, including preparing and rolling the dough and then adding the sauce and cheese. The cost of a serving of pizza (about 8 ounces) prepared from a mix was 23 to 29 cents, depending upon the brand, and was similar in cost to a serving of the refrigerated pizza. A serving of the refrigerated pizza ranged from 23 to 34 cents, depending upon the brand. Frozen pizza was generally the most expensive form; a serving ranged from 31 to 46 cents.

Meals from a Can

The same phenomenon has occurred in canned foods as in frozen foods. Manufacturers have taken the older basic products, added additional ingredients or flavorings, and built up the prices inordinately.

One of the most frequent complaints is about the small pieces of meat in canned stews and other canned meals. Consumers compare what they get with the magazine pictures of "bite-sized pieces of carefully selected beef."

We took apart a number of such products and also studied the 1969 report by the U.S. Agriculture Department for the House Consumer Subcommittee. After this investigation, I am convinced that the consumer's increasingly loud grumbling really arises from hunger pangs.

As far as "bite-sized" pieces go, it would be best to have a small mouth. We would agree that these pieces are "carefully selected." They would have to be.

There surely is "lots of rich brown gravy." The canned beef stews accurately should be called "sauce with potatoes, beef and vegetables." That is the real order of importance of their ingredients. The Agriculture Department found the two brands checked were about half sauce—an average of 48.5 percent sauce in Bounty, and 54.3 percent in Libby's.

Potatoes averaged about 23 percent in the Bounty samples and 26 percent in Libby's. Vegetables averaged 12½ percent of the contents of the Bounty beef stews and little over 4 percent in Libby's.

The actual cooked weight of the meat in the samples we

examined and those the Agriculture Department tested is about 2½ to 3½ ounces. The Agriculture Department standard requires that "canned beef stew" have at least 25 percent of beef *uncooked* weight. For a 19-ounce can this would be a minimum of 4¾ ounces. At 85 cents a pound for stew beef or boneless chuck, that means the meat in a 19-ounce can of cooked stew at 65 cents would be worth about 25 cents. We would estimate the total value of the ingredients at about 40 cents.

Bounty, at a higher cost (the equivalent of 55 cents a pound), had a higher percentage of cooked meat (18 percent) than Broadcast, at a cost of 48 cents a pound with 13 percent meat. Bounty also had a little higher percentage of meat than Libby's in the Agriculture Department tests—16.2 percent against 15.3 percent. Libby's cost per pound is about 51 cents in larger cans.

The canned beef stews do provide a little more food for the cost than brand-name frozen beef dinners. The leading brand of frozen TV dinners weighs 11 ounces. About 2¾ ounces is gravy. This leaves a little over 8 ounces of drained weight. A little over 2½ ounces is beef. In comparison, the 19-ounce canned stews have a drained weight of approximately 9-10 ounces.

The canned beef stews also are a little better value for the meat than the 8-ounce beef pot pies, unless these are on sale at less than 25 cents.

Although canned stews are more reasonable than some frozen dinners (if not necessarily satisfying in meat amount and quality), canned frankfurters and beans and meat balls and spaghetti are noticeably high-priced in comparison to the ingredients provided, and they cannot even claim to offer the relative time-saving advantage of an already prepared stew.

For example, Campbell's Beans & Franks costs 41 cents for 16 ounces. The "9 Whole Franks" are actually two inches long (some small wholes) and weigh a total of 3 ounces. In contrast, Campbell's Pork & Beans costs 17 cents for 16 ounces. After deducting the value of the beans, you pay at the rate of $1.49 for the franks.

Franco-American and Chef Boy-Ar-Dee Spaghetti with Meat Balls costs 39 cents for 15 ounces. The meat balls weigh 3 ounces. Plain canned spaghetti costs 20 cents for a 16-ounce can. So you pay 23 cents for 3 ounces of meat balls, or about $1.25 a pound. But—the cooked meat balls contain other ingredients. The actual meat content reported by the Agriculture Department was 13.3 percent, or about 2 ounces.

Granted that there is more real time-saving in prepared meat balls than in franks, the price is still high. The same is true for Spaghetti O's with eighteen Meat Balls at 41 cents for a 15½-ounce can. Plain canned Spaghetti O's are 17-19 cents at various stores. The real meat content (not including fillers to make the meat balls) is about the same as in ordinary-shaped spaghetti with meat balls. You do pay more for newer versions of spaghetti such as an "O" shape. Thus, ordinary Spaghetti with Meat Balls provides protein at a lower cost than Spaghetti O's with Meat Balls. Either gives you more protein for the money than Spaghetti O's with Sliced Franks.

In general, you get most protein for your money in ordinary canned spaghetti and cheese, followed, in order of increasing cost, by macaroni and cheese, macaroni or spaghetti and beef, Italian style spaghetti and spaghetti with meat balls.

Similarly, in canned bean products, ordinary pork and beans is the best value, followed, in order of increasing cost of the protein, by Barbecue Beans, Beef and Beans, Beans and Franks and Chili with Beans.

The table of some of the main nutrients in several leading brands of ready-to-eat products shows their cost in comparison to the nutrients provided in a serving.

Noodles and chicken in jars is costly for the small time-saving. The actual economic value of these products is a little more than half their cost, or about 28 cents compared with a product price of about 50 cents.

Nutritional Values in Soups

In soups, the differences in food values are even more extraordinary. You can pay as little as a rate of 70-80 cents for 100 grams of protein in some of the canned soups such as Split Pea with Ham and Bean with Bacon to as much as $4 to $5 for the same amount of protein in other popular varieties such as Turkey Rice, Clam Chowder and Cream of Celery.

While personal preferences, of course, dictate what you buy, all things being equal, it pays to give attention to the protein value of soups. Adults and older teens require about 60 grams of protein a day for a nutritionally adequate diet; younger teen-agers and sub-teens require about 40-50 grams; children under 10 require 25-40 grams.

The so-called "complete proteins" come from meat, poultry, fish, milk, cheese and eggs. The proteins in cereal foods are not as complete. Their nutritional value increases when they are served with a little protein from animal sources. That's why you often find ready-to-eat products have a little cheese or meat added to the spaghetti, beans or soups.

But the money-saving trick in many cases is to buy the simplest version and add the additional small amount of meat or other animal protein yourself. That way you get maximum nutrition at lowest cost, while still getting most of the convenience.

Because of the desirability of buying the most protein for your money, here is a report on several of the best (and worst) buys in protein and other nutrients in canned soups. You can't judge the food value by the price. Some of the lower-priced soups have relatively little nutrition; some have more.

We based our comparison on the nutritional analysis of the most widely-sold brand, Campbell's. But the growing number of private-brand canned soups such as Co-op and Ann Page can be assumed to have similar relative values. Thus, vegetable beef usually would be higher in protein and cheaper in protein cost than plain vegetable, etc.

Nor did we attempt to compare food values among different brands, although the private-brand soups we priced usually were 2 to 6 cents less than the national brands.

Some of the canned soups are good buys in protein, providing as much as a third or more of the nutritionally desirable protein for a meal.

The best nutritional buy we found in any canned soup is Split Pea with Ham. It provides protein at a cost per 100 grams of 72 cents, and is high in other nutrients.

Others of the relatively better buys, in order of increasing cost of the protein, are: Bean with Bacon (83 cents per 100 grams); Green Pea (92 cents); Beef (96 cents); Hot Dog Bean (99 cents);

Chicken Broth ($1.21); Pepper Pot ($1.36); Chicken 'n Dumpling ($1.43); Turkey Noodle ($1.44); Vegetable Beef ($1.47); Consomme ($1.63); Vegetable and Beef Stockpot ($1.63); Scotch Broth ($1.67); Chicken & Stars ($1.96); Beef Broth ($2.04); Vegetable ($2.10); Chicken Vegetable ($2.16); Onion ($2.19); Minestrone ($2.22); Noodles and Ground Beef ($2.22); Chicken Noodle ($2.22); Beef Noodle ($2.29).

This is not to say that all of the others are nutritionally low. It just means they may be costlier for the protein and some of the other nutrients provided. Nor are those that are inexpensive for the protein provided necessarily always the highest nutritionally. Most are. But Vegetable Soup, for example, while only moderate in the protein provided, is one of the lowest in price. Turkey Noodle is no richer in protein than Chicken & Stars, but usually costs less. (Anytime food manufacturers make noodles into a different shape they want extra pay for it.)

The worst buys in protein value in canned soups are usually the so-called "cream" soups: Cream of Asparagus, Cream of Potato, Cream of Celery, etc. The tomato soups also are relatively poor buys in protein, even though usually lowest priced.

The new canned soups with water already added apparently are intended to solve one of the least difficult cooking chores yet discovered, that of adding water to condensed soups. We found the price equally watered. These products also show how little you may get of a key ingredient, such as the turkey in turkey soup.

A can of condensed Turkey Noodle Soup costs you 18 cents. A can of Great American Tasty Turkey Noodle costs you 25 cents. Draining the liquid from both, we found the prewatered soup had about 6½ ounces of solids, mostly noodles and rice. These included two small chunks and some slivers, bits and pieces of meat. My wife, who with Elaine Jessen, my research assistant, tweezered out the two small chunks and remaining slivers and bits of turkey, wants you to know that they gave the manufacturer the benefit of every doubt. The total turkey they could rescue weighed a half ounce.

The cheaper condensed soup had 5¾ ounces of solids, including three-eighths of an ounce of turkey.

But now Campbell's is competing both with itself and Heinz with its own prewatered Chunky Soups. The Chunky turkey variety, with a 57-cent price tag for 18 ¾ ounces, is exactly three times the price of Campbell's Turkey Noodle Soup, and has just 10 ½ ounces of solids, including 1 ½ ounces of turkey. The other solids were rather nice looking potatoes and other vegetables, flavorings and the omnipresent caramel coloring.

The prewatered soups have drawn fire from some of the more alert shoppers. A Colorado Springs lawyer wrote to Heinz, reporting on his own comparison of the company's "don't dilute" Cream of Mushroom Soup with a can of Heinz Condensed Cream of Mushroom. For 25 cents for the already diluted soup he got 14 ¾ ounces. For the 15 cents he paid for the condensed soup, he got 21 ounces (10 ½-ounce can plus one can of water). "I found the ingredients and the taste virtually identical," he told the manufacturer. "It seems you are either selling the water in the Great American Soups at the rate of $1.20 a gallon or have raised the price for cream of mushroom soup by 230 percent merely by changing the package."

At the Zurich conference on processed foods in 1968, an economist, Dr. W. Wyss of Lucerne, reported that one of the problems manufacturers had to overcome was "the Gretchen complex." This is the guilt feeling some housewives have who think that they are not fulfilling their family duty when they buy ready-to-eat foods instead of doing their own cooking.

Lipton uses psychologically hip TV commercials to reassure any guilt-feeling housewives. No doubt you have seen these commercials. They show youngsters calling into the house, "Is it soup yet?" The announcer then says, "We only supply the ingredients, you do the cooking." Mama is shown intently stirring a pot and peering and sniffing at it as though she really were cooking soup instead of pretend-cooking a dried soup mixture.

But this TV Gretchen at least did add the water.

MAJOR INGREDIENTS IN LEADING MEAT AND POULTRY PRODUCTS*

Product	Unit Cost	Stated Net Weight**	Meat Weight	% Meat	% Potato	% Noodles, Spaghetti or Macaroni	% Vegetables	% Sauce
Bounty Beef Stew	65¢	19 oz.	3.1 oz.	16.2%	22.9%		12.5%	48.5%
Libby's Beef Stew	45	15	2.3	15.3	26.3		4.2	54.3
College Inn Egg Noodles and Chicken	50	16	1.6	9.9		67.1%		23.0
Derby Egg Noodles and Chicken	n.a.	14¾	1.6	10.8		65.4		23.8
Chef Boy-Ar-Dee Beefaroni	39	15	1.3	8.5		48.3		43.2
Chef Boy-Ar-Dee Spaghetti and Meat Balls	39	15	2.0	13.3		49.9		36.8
Franco-American Spaghetti w/Meat Balls	39	15	2.05	13.3		28.9		57.8
Franco-American Macaroni 'n Beef in Tomato Sauce	32	15	1.4	9.3		45.1		45.6
Heinz Beef Stew	n.a.	8½	1.45	17.2	20.8		12.2	51.6
Chef Boy-Ar-Dee Beef-O-Getti	39	15	2.5	16.7		32.3		51.0
Franco-American Spaghetti O's w/18 Little Meat Balls	41	15	2.1	14.0		46.9		39.1
Armour Chopped Beef	n.a.	12	11.1	92.6				7.4

*From tests made by U. S. Agriculture Dept., 1969, for House Consumer Subcommittee. Results are averages of two to four samples for each product.

**This is net weight as shown on label. Actual weight may differ; most often was a little higher than stated weight.

COMPARATIVE NUTRIENTS IN CANNED READY-TO-EAT FOODS
Nutrients per Serving*

	Ounces	Unit Price	Protein	Calcium	Iron	Vit.A	Thiamine	Riboflavin	Niacin
Campbell's									
Barbecue Beans	16 oz.	29¢	5.7	60	2.4	255	.08	.06	0.6
Beans & Franks in Tomato Sauce	16	41	8.4	63	2.4	128	.06	.06	1.1
Beans 'n Beef in Tomato Sauce	16	33	7.1	74	2.6	860	.07	.05	1.8
Pork & Beans w/Tomato Sauce	16	17	7.1	52	2.1	113	.06	.04	0.8
" " " "	21	23	7.1	52	2.1	113	.06	.04	0.8
Bounty									
Chili Con Carne w/Beans	15¾	39	7.0	31	1.9	583	.05	.07	2.2
Corned Beef Hash	15½	53	9.8	15	2.0	trace	.01	.03	2.1
Franco-American									
Beef Gravy	10¾	21	5.2	10	1.0	trace	.04	.05	1.2
Giblet Gravy	10¾	21	1.8	9	0.9	490	.03	.03	0.3
Chicken Gravy	10½	21	2.3	11	1.0	583	.01	.05	0.7
Mushroom Gravy	10½	21	1.6	trace	0.3	trace	trace	.06	0.7
Spaghetti Sauce w/Meat	15½	33	4.6	13	1.8	2614	.04	.06	1.3
Italian Style Spaghetti	15¼	25	3.5	24	0.8	255	.09	.05	1.1
Macaroni 'n Beef in Tomato Sauce	15	32	5.4	21	0.6	353	.16	.08	2.2
Macaroni & Cheese	15	25	3.7	56	0.6	228	.09	.09	1.2
Macaroni O's w/Cheese Sauce	15	29	3.4	57	0.9	270	.12	.14	0.8
Spaghetti in Tomato Sauce w/Cheese	15¼	21	3.2	16	0.8	200	.14	.10	1.4
Spaghetti 'n Beef in Tomato Sauce	15	33	4.9	11	1.0	750	.17	.08	2.3
Spaghetti w/Meat Balls	15	39	4.9	9	1.0	485	.08	.08	1.6
Spaghetti O's in Tomato and Cheese Sauce	26	33	2.7	25	0.6	350	.10	.09	1.4
Spaghetti O's w/Meat Balls	15	41	4.7	25	0.7	425	.14	.09	1.4
Spaghetti O's w/Sliced Franks	15	39	3.9	23	0.5	280	.13	.09	1.5

*Servings are as suggested by the manufacturer. Protein value is in grams; other nutrients in milligrams, except Vitamin A (International Units).

CHAPTER

4

THE MODERN WOMAN'S BAG:
A CONVENIENCE COOKING POUCH

The American woman who thinks she has at last found her bag in the shape of a convenience cooking pouch often is only boiling away her money, without saving any real time.

By extensive advertising, and because of the gullibility of the average consumer, packers are able to charge almost two or three times as much for ordinary frozen vegetables if they add a few additional ingredients and some minor cooking convenience—sometimes so minor it is virtually non-existent.

In our surveys we have found, for example, plain frozen peas in a 2-pound pour bag selling for 26 cents a pound; in a 10-ounce package the cost per pound becomes 33 cents; with a little sauce added and packaged in a pouch the price is 66 cents; and, finally, with rice and mushrooms added, the cost is 94 cents a pound.

In making these criticisms, I do not want to detract from the values of frozen produce. In general, they have provided some real convenience and have made available a greater variety of foods out of season. To some extent but not always or to a really significant degree, frozen produce has higher nutritional value and better flavor than canned fruits and vegetables, although rarely as much as fresh foods.

But a great deal of exaggeration also has developed. One is the myth of superior nutrition. Often claims are made by freezer salesmen in the U.S. and sometimes by the frozen-food industry, that frozen foods provide better nutrition even than fresh foods prepared at home, let alone canned foods.

Among the reasons sometimes claimed for the superiority of frozen foods are the long distances fresh produce travels to market, and poor cooking methods in the home. The criticized cooking habits include cooking a long time, using too much water, and then throwing out this liquid, which may have up to half the vitamin value. Some of these claims are but grains of truth which have been exaggerated. The one point that may have wide validity is that poor cooking habits often rob families of some of their vitamins.

But the claim that fresh produce loses nutritional value because of shipping long distances and poor store handling may be as true for frozen foods as for fresh.

While frozen foods often are described as superior in nutrition and flavor because they are frozen at the peak of ripeness, the fact is, they can suffer loss of value on the way to and in the stores. They can thaw and be refrozen at any of several points.

On a number of occasions, I have seen thawed packages of frozen foods among the top layers in the freezer cabinets of supermarkets. This happens because the stock clerks pile packages above the frost line. Then when the cabinets are defrosted the top packages thaw, and subsequently are refrozen.

In frozen vegetables, this may merely result in some loss of flavor and nutrition but the food may still be edible. The U.S. Agriculture Department says that frozen fruits and vegetables and red meats *can* be refrozen if they have been held at refrigerator temperatures for no more than a few days, and if they appear in good condition. But with frozen precooked foods the problem can be more serious, as discussed in Chapter 13.

(In this connection, it is best to buy frozen foods at the end of shopping, to ask the clerk to put frozen foods in an insulated or double paper bag, to avoid delay in getting home with them, and to rotate the contents of the freezer compartment, using the oldest foods first.)

In the absence of any legal safeguard, the consumer is unable to tell if frozen foods have been adequately protected until she opens the package. Consumers usually try to make sure packages are hard-frozen by squeezing them. This, of course, is no assurance. A frozen-food package feels as solid at twenty degrees Fahrenheit as at zero. But at twenty degrees the quality, including the vitamin value, can decline even in one day. Nor can the quality be restored by reducing the temperature to zero, although further damage can be prevented.

Only when you open the package may you realize, from the loss of color, or large amount of frost inside the package, or changes in texture or flavor, that the produce has suffered temperature damage.

Assuming reasonable care in processing and handling, in general you can expect almost as high nutritional value in frozen vegetables and fruits as in fresh, and a little higher nutritional level than in canned. As one example, 100 grams (3½ ounces) of frozen green beans, one of the most popular frozen vegetables, after cooking and draining provide 5 milligrams of vitamin C, compared with 12 for fresh, and 4 for canned; 580 milligrams of vitamin A, compared with 540 for fresh, and 290 for canned; somewhat less protein than fresh but more than canned; less iron, although a little more calcium, than canned.[7]

These comparisons assume you use the liquid in canned vegetables in one way or another, as you should, since it has some of the nutrients you paid for.

Other comparisons of food values of popular frozen, fresh and canned produce items are shown in the table in this chapter. Especially noteworthy is the high nutritional value of frozen orange juice concentrate, one of the most useful frozen foods because it is one of the few that actually is as high nutritionally as the fresh equivalent, and yet costs less. But frozen foods usually are not as good economic value as either the fresh equivalent in season or the canned equivalent, even taking into account the lower nutritional value of the canned items. There is a serious question of how much extra you should be willing to pay for a little more nutritional value.

The really controversial group of frozen foods that has become a money trap for unwary buyers is frozen precooked foods, many of which were discussed in Chapter 3.

Similarly, the frozen fruit pies have much less nutritional value than standard home recipes. This is not too surprising, considering the small amount of fruit and large amount of fillers

used in the frozen pies. Frozen cherry pie has about 20 percent
less iron, only about two-thirds of the vitamin A, and also less of
other important nutrients.

The Food and Drug Administration and packers even have
battled over how many cherries a frozen cherry pie should have.
Consumers complained because the pictures on the packages
showed pies brimming over with cherries, but when they cut into
such pies they found a lot less fruit than the pictures had led
them to expect. As an example of the difficulty of setting
standards, the FDA proposal to establish a minimum standard
of 2.7 cherries per ounce found sharp resistance from the
packers.

Usually a 10-ounce package of a frozen vegetable yields
almost the same amount of cooked vegetable as a 16-ounce can
of that vegetable. Here are some examples provided by Virginia
McLuckie, Maryland State extension food economist:

COMPARATIVE YIELDS OF COOKED FOOD

	Fresh	Frozen	Canned
Asparagus	47%	93%	63%
Green Beans	94	91	49
Lima Beans	37	100	60
Broccoli Spears	69	85	––
Brussels Sprouts	79	96	62
Whole-Kernel Corn	44	97	61
Green Peas	38	85	58
Spinach	60	77	51
Candied Sweet Potatoes	84	100	63

Thus when 10-ounce packages of popular frozen vegetables such as green peas or corn cost a little less or at least no more than the 16-ounce canned versions they are approximately as good value, taste preference aside. Supermarket sales of their own brand frozen vegetables are sometimes less in cost than the canned versions. The private-brand 2-pound and 1½-pound pour bags especially can be remarkable values and are actually more convenient than the 10-ounce packages, since you can pour out just the amount you need and close the bag again.

But the cost problem arises with the addition of other ingredients such as a sauce, or the blending of several foods, all in a boilable pouch, at a disproportionately higher price.

Green Giant Rice Verdi, labeled "rice with bell peppers and parsley" costs you 41 cents in a 12-ounce package. It represents mainly about 5 ounces of instant uncooked rice, worth 13 cents. The other ingredients, in order of importance, are margarine, green peppers, salt, chicken bouillon flavoring, cornstarch, onion flakes and parsley flakes.

Curiously, the rice in the boilable pouch actually takes longer to cook—16 minutes as against 7 minutes for ordinary rice.

Or take French-cut string beans. Plain frozen string beans are available for as little as 22 cents in a 9-ounce package. With a butter sauce the price rises to 31 cents. But with a few sautéed mushrooms, the price becomes 39 cents.

If a packer mixes together several different frozen vegetables, adds a sauce and a glamorous international name such as Parisian Style Vegetables, Bavarian Style, Mexican Style and so on, you may find that you pay as much for the sauce as for the vegetables. We estimated that the value of the carrots, celery, onion and mushrooms in the Parisian Style frozen vegetables was about 21 cents, in comparison to the 45-cent price of the 10-ounce package. Almost half of the package contents were raw carrots, worth 5 cents. The most expensive ingredient was about 12 cents worth of sliced mushrooms.

Similarly, the Japanese Style Vegetables had about 24 cents worth of ingredients with French-style green beans most prominent.

Even similar pre-seasoned canned vegetables cost much less. Ordinary canned mixed vegetables yield many of the same vegetables as Mexican Style frozen vegetables at less than half the cost. Canned zucchini squash has the same leading ingredient as the Frozen Spanish Style Vegetable Medley, plus lots of flavoring, at one-third less cost.

Apparently many women do not stop to weigh small conveniences against large added costs. First introduced in 1961, in the four years from 1965 to 1968 sales of boil-in-pouch jumped almost 60 percent.

The entire trend of the brand-name packers is toward still more combinations of vegetables and sauce in throw-away cooking materials. The giant of the boil-in-a-bag industry, in fact the Green Giant, by 1970 already was selling twenty-four different kinds of frozen vegetables in butter, cream or cheese sauces. Already on the market as this is written are frozen vegetables in an aluminum pan for range-top heating, and frozen vegetable casseroles packaged in an oven film. On the way are boil-in-a-tray vegetables.[8] (Cooking in your own pan not only saves you money, but your own pan can be recycled.)

Another promotion is for supposedly quicker-cooking frozen vegetables: for example, "five-minute" vegetables. This turns out to be five minutes of simmering *after* bringing to a boil— much the same time as for ordinary frozen vegetables, with a small difference in cooking method.

Illusions of Value

In fresh and canned fruits and vegetables, too, there are illusions of value.

Many people pay higher prices for produce because of prettier or more perfect appearance. Red-skinned apples are priced almost according to the amount of red. The redder they are, the more they cost, the U.S. Agriculture Department's Consumer and Marketing Service points out. But there is little difference in the taste.

Similarly, oranges with greenish skins and grapefruit with rust-colored splotches cost less, but may be of average or superior quality inside. Perfectly round onions command a higher price than those that are lopsided.

Large sizes of fruits and vegetables sometimes also command an extra price. But they are not always the best quality, let alone the most economical.

In prunes, for example, the difference in edible yield is less than 10 percent between the large and small sizes. Yet the small sizes sometimes cost 30-40 percent less.

In either frozen or canned vegetables, whole vegetables, such as whole beans or asparagus, cost more than cut styles, not for any added food value but merely because it is harder for packers to keep these fragile vegetables whole during processing, the *1969 Yearbook of Agriculture* points out. Diced, short cuts or pieces of vegetables all cost less. In fact, short cut beans, even though they cost less, yield slightly more beans in the can than do French style, whole cuts or cuts longer than 1 ½ inches.

In canned fruits, the main difference between fruits in "heavy" syrup and the cheaper "light" syrup is less than an ounce of sugar. Too, the lower-priced canned fruits and vegetables may be irregular-shaped pieces, not the uniform pieces of the costlier brands. The nutritional value is exactly the same.

The Shopping Roulette of Canned Goods

One of the most bitter complaints from consumers is the amount of liquid in cans of fruits and vegetables and what seems to be a relatively low yield, especially sometimes of fruit.

The government sets a minimum fill for the drained net weight. But some packers give more solid food above the minimum and less liquid than others. Unfortunately, under present circumstances the only way to know is through trial—always an expensive process. The government has been urged to require that packers show on the label the actual drained weight as well as the total net weight.

But the Food and Drug Administration, which could require this disclosure, responded to our inquiry in October, 1970, with a comment that it had no plan at that time for such a requirement. At congressional hearings, the House Consumer Subcommittee staff had shown the differences between contents and the amount of liquid. But the FDA representative at that time had argued that the liquid had food value. The canning industry itself is vigorously resisting.

There are admitted problems of control which make exact uniformity of fill impossible. But at the same time consumers are really buying such products for their solid content and sometimes find using all the liquid a problem in resourcefulness.

A summary of the comparative drained weights of several brands and types of canned vegetables demonstrated at the House hearings is shown in the table in this chapter. One fact that is noticeable is that price is not necessarily a criterion; the lower-priced private brands offer much the same solid content as the higher-priced advertised brands. We found this to be true in our own tests with advertised and private brands of canned peas (see Chapter 16).

The Consumers' Association of Canada also found the amount of fill did not depend on whether the brand was advertised or private. In 14-ounce cans of green beans the amount of solids ranged from 7 to 9 ounces in most brands. What the CAC did find was that in all brands some cans were not the labeled 14 ounces, but only 12. In canned peaches the association concluded that often the best buy is simply the cheapest brand. Price was no indication of either quantity or quality.[9]

Several value guides can be gleaned from the table of comparative drained weights:

—The size of cans of whole-kernel corn is not necessarily indicative of their content. The 12-ounce vacuum pack with its low liquid content yields virtually as much drained weight as the brine-packed 16- and 17-ounce cans. At their lower price, vacuum packs are a better value. But if you also use the liquid, as in a soup or chowder, the brine pack would be better value. The liquid has some of the milk of the corn.

—In canned fruits, sliced pineapple provides more actual fruit and is priced lowest. You pay at the rate of 32 cents a pound for solid content. Fruit cocktail and peaches are better value than pears, with a cost per pound of 39 to 40 cents. Canned pears, with the lowest actual content and higher prices, have a cost per pound, in this sampling, of 58 cents.

—The importance of using the liquid in both vegetables and fruits cannot be overstressed. Vitamin C and other vitamins in these precooked products are water soluble. The liquid in canned vegetables usually contains about 40 percent of the vitamin C and one-fourth to one-third of the thiamine and riboflavin (B vitamins). The liquid can be boiled down to make a sauce for the vegetable or for use in soups, gravies and other dishes.

The percentage of vitamins contained in the liquid is even greater in canned fruits—as much as half in some varieties and at least one-third in most.

While this information can make you alert to the values in canned produce and conscious of the amount of fill, the shopping-roulette problem will not really be lessened until the Food and Drug Administration moves to require the statement of drained weight on the label, and until the Agriculture Department is less permissive in the level of its standards for fill. For example, a standard for canned peas and carrots announced in 1970 requires only about 68 percent drained weight, and the standard for fruit cocktail, only 65 percent. Many of the standards for fruit require only amounts "which can be sealed without crushing or breaking," thus leaving much to the canner's judgment.

There also are questions as to whether the factors used in quality grading are always geared to consumer needs—for example, whether there is excessive emphasis on appearance in Grade A, and excessive permission for moisture in Grade C. That is why I have suggested that the second grade, called U.S. Grade B or U.S. Standard, usually is the best value.

COMPARING NUTRITIONAL VALUES, 100 GRAMS, OF FROZEN FOODS*

	Vit. C	*Vit. A*
Orange juice, raw (Fla.)	45 mg.	200 I.U.
Canned, unsweetened	40	200
Frozen, concentrate	45	200
Crystals, water added	44	200
Peaches, raw	7	1,330
Canned (solids, liquid)	4	440
Frozen, sliced, sweetened	11	650

	Vit. C	Vit. A
Pineapple, fresh	17 mg.	70 I.U.
Canned, incl. syrup	7	50
Canned, juice pack	10	60
Frozen chunks, sweetened	8	30
Pineapple juice, canned	9	10
Frozen, reconstituted	12	50

	Vit. C	Calcium	Vit. A	Protein	Iron
Peas, fresh (cooked, drained)	20 mg.	23 mg.	540 I.U.	5.4 gm.	1.8 mg.
Canned (incl. liquid)	9	19	450	3.4	1.5
Frozen (cooked, drained)	13	19	600	5.1	1.9
Spinach (cooked, drained)	28	93	8,100	3	2.2
Canned (incl. liquid)	14	85	5,500	2.7	2.1
Frozen (cooked, drained)	28	105	8,100	2.9	2.5

Ready-to-Eat Foods

	Protein	Calcium	Phosphorus	Vit. A
Chicken pot pie				
Home prepared	10.1 gm.		100 mg.	1,330 I.U.
Frozen heat-and-serve	6.7		50	910
Fish Cakes				
Home prepared	14.7			
Frozen heat-and-serve	9.2			
Pies				
Coconut Custard				
Home prepared	6	94 mg.		230
Frozen	6	95		160
Cherry				
Home prepared	2.6	14		440
Frozen	2.2	12		290
Apple				
Home prepared	2.2	8		30
Frozen	1.9	8		10

*100 grams equals 3½ ounces.

COMPARATIVE DRAINED WEIGHTS*

	Avg. Net Weight	Avg. Drained Weight	Avg. Unit Price
Asparagus, spears			39¢
Del Monte (14½ oz.)	15.7 oz.	9.4 oz.	
Town House (14 oz.)	15.3	9.6	
Ritter (13 oz.)	13.2	8.5	
Beets, sliced			20
Del Monte (16 oz.)	16.7	10.5	
Corn, whole kernel (12 oz.)			22
Del Monte	13.3	10.9	
Green Giant	12.8	10.7	
Highway	12.6	10.9	
Corn, whole kernel			25
Del Monte (17 oz.)	17.1	11.2	
Silver Run (16 oz.)	16.7	11.1	
Town House (16 oz.)	17.6	11.4	
Dill pickles, slices (32 oz.)			49
Heinz	34.2	20.7	
Zippy	34.0	20.5	
Green Beans, cut (16 oz.)			22
Del Monte	16.6	9.7	
Town House	16.5	9.7	
Hanover (glass)	16.5	10.3	
Mushrooms, sliced			33
B in B (broiled in butter, 3 oz.)	5.5	3.3	
Green Giant (2½ oz.)	4.1	2.7	
Peas, mixed sizes			29
Town House (16 oz.)	17.3	10.6	
Del Monte (17 oz.)	17.5	11.5	
Green Giant (17 oz.)	17.6	11.4	
Spinach, whole leaf			20
Town House (15 oz.)	16.4	11.6	

	Avg. Net Weight	Avg. Drained Weight	Avg. Unit Price
Fruit Cocktail			29¢
Town House (16 oz.)	17.1 oz.	11.9 oz.	
Del Monte (17 oz.)	17.6	11.9	
Grapefruit, sections (16 oz.)			29
Town House	17.5	10.2	
Del Monte	17.4	10.6	
Peaches, sliced (16 oz.)			28
Town House	17.2	11.3	
Del Monte	17.3	11.4	
Peaches, halves (16 oz.)**			28
Town House	17.3	11.5	
Del Monte	17.4	11.3	
Pears, halves (16 oz.)**			34
Town House	16.7	9.3	
Del Monte	17.0	9.4	
Pineapple, chunk (20 oz.)			35
Dole	20.7	13.6	
Del Monte	21.3	13.8	
Pineapple, sliced (20½ oz.)			29
La Lani	21.3	14.0	

---

*Adapted from tests by U. S. Agriculture Department for House Consumer Sub-committee, 1969.

**Count of canned peach halves ranged from 5 to 8, most often 5 or 6. On pear halves, count was 5 or 6 to a can. Number of halves did not affect drained weight materially. A higher count usually indicated slightly smaller fruit.

CHAPTER

5

THE WAR OVER YOUR
CEREAL BOWL

Ready-to-eat cereals have become one of the most frequent family money leaks and nutritional concerns. Ready-to-eat cereals usually cost about twice as much per serving as cereals you cook yourself. Nor do they provide as much nourishment per serving. A 1-ounce serving of oatmeal costs about a penny and a half and yields 4 grams of protein. A similar serving of cornflakes costs 2½ cents and yields a little over 2 grams, and also less of other nutrients.

But even among dry cereals, each added convenience costs you disproportionately more. Ordinary quick-rolled oats, which cook in one minute, cost you only 1.5 cents an ounce. Buy oats in the form of Cheerios or Frosty-O's, a "sugar charged" oat cereal, and you pay 3½ cents an ounce. Buy it in the form of Kellogg's Froot Loops, which is sugared and fruit-flavored oat cereal, and you pay 5 cents an ounce. Actually, since the leading ingredient in Froot Loops is sugar, with oat flour second, you pay about 6 cents an ounce for the oat flour and other nonsugar nutrients.

If packed in individual serving boxes, cereals cost 70 to 100 percent more than in the large boxes. If you calculate the real cost, you pay as much as $1.15 a pound for these individual servings.

A glaring example of "convenience" that really is no

convenience at all is the higher cost of even the same cereal in premeasured packets for individual servings. Like many modern packaging "innovations," this pseudo-convenience is more accurately a money-waster and pollution-maker. As the table of hot cereal costs shows, you pay about 46 percent more for the same Instant H-O Oatmeal in premeasured paper packets —about a nickel more for four servings. Similarly, you pay 100 percent more for the same Instant Hot Ralston in premeasured packets—about 9 cents more for four servings. We did not bother to measure the time required to pour the wanted number of servings into a measuring cup and to rinse it out. Convenience-lovers may also be interested to know that a tablespoon is a handy measuring device and can be used over and over.

There really are four basic cereal grains commonly used to manufacture breakfast cereals: corn, rice, wheat and oats. (Barley also is sometimes used.) But manufacturers have made so many different versions that, as noted in Chapter 1, in a typical supermarket you can count eighty different types. The original cereals are flaked or puffed in size; made in different shapes such as O's, alphabet letters, animals, biscuits or crowns; flavored with sugar, cocoa, fruit flavorings and bits of marshmallow and other ingredients.

In the manufacturing process the original cereals lose even some of the vitamin value through the exploding, puffing, flaking and toasting they undergo.

In recent years the puffed cereals have been even more puffed up as the result of new processes for exploding grains of wheat and rice to a greater volume than previously had been the practice. That is why the packages of modern puffed rice and puffed wheat look so large—two or three times the size of the same amount of more compact cereals. Never have so many people bought so little food in such big boxes.

Many of the new versions even have lost their original identification and are promoted under such invented names as Cap'n Crunch, Froot Loops, Kaboom, Life, Total, Product 19 and so on. Thus, value comparisons are even harder for the already confused consumer.

The main drive of the cereal manufacturers has been to

capture the children's market through heavy TV advertising and premiums, and equally heavy sweetening of the product itself. (The three largest cereal manufacturers in 1970 spent over $40 million advertising breakfast cereals on TV, mainly to children. Their domination of the cereal business has led to an investigation by the FTC, now in progress, seeking to assess whether such pervasive advertising has established, in effect, a monopoly and raised prices.) Some products, while called "oat cereals," actually have as much or more sugar than oatmeal, as shown in the list of ingredients on the package. It might be more accurate to call Froot Loops and Kaboom, for example, oat-flavored candies, since sugar is their leading ingredient.

Not only are the sugared cereals more expensive, but they are nutritionally inferior to even the plain ready-to-eat cereals on which children have to sprinkle the sugar themselves, as the table at the end of this chapter shows. Sugar-frosted or other presweetened corn flakes usually have about 33 percent additional sugar, or almost 3½ ounces in the case of a 10-ounce package costing 38 cents. Since the remaining 6½ ounces of enriched cornflakes can be bought in their plain version for about 20 cents, you are, in effect, paying 18 cents for the sugar or at the rate of 90 cents a pound. Sugar, of course, is worth about 13 cents a pound at the retail counter.

The nutritional inferiority of the presweetened cereals is shown in the table. A 1-ounce serving of ordinary cornflakes has about 2 grams of protein; of presweetened cornflakes only about 1.2 grams. The ordinary cornflakes also have about 50 percent more iron, twice as much calcium and almost twice as much of the B vitamins. Similarly, plain puffed wheat has two and a half times as much protein and more of the other significant nutrients than sugared puffed wheat.

Revealingly, most of the cereals promoted on children's TV programs are the relatively low-nutrition but higher-priced presweetened and flavored types, often advertised with unmerited implications of powerful nutrition.

The wide range between the economic value of the original cereal grain and the manufactured dry cereal is shown by the fact that an ounce of uncooked dry rice costs about a penny, and an ounce of puffed rice costs almost 6 cents. Yet the ounce of uncooked rice can provide about twice as much protein and more calcium, iron and thiamine than the ounce of puffed rice, Dr. Michael C. Latham, Cornell University Professor of International Nutrition, has pointed out.

While cereal promotion has been aimed most heavily at children, the newest promotional tack of the large manufacturers is vitamin fortification, with the introduction of such brands as Total, Life, Product 19 and others. These are really the equivalent of a basic cereal with a vitamin pill (or capsule)—in fact, a rather cheap vitamin pill, richer in the cheap vitamins but lower in the relatively costly B vitamins. I estimate the value of the added vitamins in a serving at 1 to 2 cents if bought in pill or capsule form.

Between the confusing nomenclature and packaging of some of the fortified cereals, and well-intended but misinterpreted Senate hearings in 1970, the public has become noticeably bewildered about the nutritional value of these and other ready-to-eat cereals. After the hearings such comments from consumers were heard as, "Those cereals have no nutrition at all." "I buy Total, the one that has nutrition." At the same time newspaper writers made such off-hand remarks as, "Cereal has about as much nutrition as dirty fingernails. . . ."

Contributing to the confusion were (1) a public-spirited engineer-turned-nutritionist named Robert Choate, who had a good deal of truth on his side but whose comments on TV ads were overshadowed by his nutritional criticism; (2) a well-meaning but inexperienced Senate staff, which brought up the problem but failed to put it into proper perspective; (3) the cereal manufacturers and their spokesmen, who jumped on the minor flaws in Choate's testimony about cereals at the Senate hearings and really confused the issue with a smokescreen of sophistry; and (4) the newspapers and TV stations, which sensationalized the controversy without investigating further to find the answers, or providing reliable guidance.

It was notably unfair to raise these issues and then leave consumers worried and bewildered.

Choate was perfectly right in criticizing widely used dry cereals for their exaggerated TV advertising, aimed especially at children, and for their inflated prices.

But what confused the issue were his ratings of cereals on their content of nine nutrients, including some such as vitamins C, D and A that you ordinarily don't expect cereals to supply and which are normally supplied by other foods. He gave equal weight to these "cheap" vitamins and the costlier protein and B vitamins. On the basis of this kind of classification, Choate's ratings ranked especially high the fortified cereals with added vitamins.

Actually, of course, most reasonably balanced daily diets which include fruit juices, vegetables, milk and other dairy products do not require these added vitamins. An excess of some vitamins such as A and D can be harmful, or merely wasted, as in the case of larger amounts of vitamin C than the body can absorb. The fortified breakfast cereals command a higher price than many other common breakfast foods and for the most part provide only some additional synthetic vitamins and in some cases a little extra protein.

It would be more useful to rate cereals on the basis of the B vitamins and iron that nutritionists usually expect them to supply toward your total nutritional intake, and also on the calcium and moderate amount of protein (the really expensive and valuable nutrient) they supply.

Vitamin-pill manufacturers immediately sought to capitalize on fears aroused by the oversimplified characterization of ordinary cereals as "empty calories" by advertising that families should take a multi-vitamin pill every day to make sure.

The even more serious problem is that people can be led to assume that a fortified cereal supplies more nourishment than it actually does. You or your child may assume more from the name or the advertising than the cereal provides. Total is not at all a total food. As the table shows, it is relatively low in protein and even with 4 ounces of milk will not provide the desirable 15 to 20 grams for breakfast. Nor will Team make your son an athlete. It too is relatively low in protein. Kaboom does not even list its protein content but in general presugared cereals are low in protein, as the table shows. Incidentally, Special K, advertised for watching weight, actually has somewhat more calories than some of the cereals not so advertised.

Nor is the protein in breakfast cereals as complete as

proteins from animal sources. The protein in milk, which usually is used with dry cereal, does, of course, supplement cereal protein.

But the cereal manufacturers and their defenders were the ones who really muddied the waters. For example, Dr. Frederick J. Stare, a Harvard nutritionist who often defends food processors, retorted that Choate's testimony ignored the fact that "95 percent of breakfast cereals are consumed with milk."

If milk is the main nutritional value in eating dry cereals, then obviously there are easier ways to drink it than with a spoon.

Even more misleading was the rebuttal to Choate by a Quaker Oats Co. official to the effect that if milk were added to the cereals, they would all have more food value than an egg, a slice of bread or a number of other common breakfast foods. This is really kidding the public.

It is the milk, of course, that really fortifies the cereal. Without the milk a 1-ounce serving of cornflakes has a protein efficiency rating of 234 (determined by relating protein quality and quantity) compared with 850 for one egg. The milk itself has a rating of 518. Even a 1-ounce serving of fortified oat flakes has a rating for itself of only 436.

For years the cereal industry has showered teachers, home economists and newspaper writers with promotional literature. It is time to set the record straight on some of these widespread promotion claims fed through the teachers and writers to the public.

The industry claim: "Different kinds of cereals vary in price according to their convenience, ingredients and nutrients. Few foods, for such low cost, can provide the nutritional value, variety and taste appeal that you get for your money in a serving of cereal and milk."

The facts: Prices of ready-to-eat cereals vary more in accordance with the amount of money spent to advertise them. This is shown by the sharply lower cost of the private brands and by the fact that the best-selling packaged cereals have the highest advertising cost (usually 20 percent of the price you pay, one government study found). Nor are they cheaper than other usual breakfast foods, as demonstrated in the "bargain" argument below.

The claim: "Many new and interesting breakfast cereals have been created for the benefit of consumers and better breakfasts. [They] bring added convenience and nutritional values. . ."

The facts: The National Commission on Food Marketing found that new versions are continuously introduced to stimulate consumer interest, especially that of the child consumers. Cereals of the presweetened kind actually reduce nutritional values.

The claim: "You have a breakfast bargain."

The facts: As the table shows, many other common breakfast foods, such as eggs, toast, muffins, pancakes and so on are cheaper and often nutritionally superior.

Here are other facts which may help to clarify the breakfast controversy:

—The most nutritionally complete breakfast for the money would be an egg or a little meat other than bacon (primarily a fat), a slice or two of bread and a half-cup or more of milk, assuming you get vitamin C in your meal in the form of juice. (A really inexpensive breakfast, Choate suggests, would be rice pudding and reconstituted nonfat milk.)

—If you prefer cereal, cooked cereals not only cost less but provide somewhat more nutrition than dry cereals. A little of the original nutritive value of grains and cereals is lost in manufacturing ready-to-eat cereals. Of the cooked cereals, oatmeal has the most protein.

—If you don't have even the one minute needed to cook a cereal, a slice of bread or muffin with some milk is the equivalent, at less expense, of the ready-to-eat cereals.

—If you prefer a ready-to-eat cereal, then buy the least expensive private brand, and preferably a whole-grain cereal. For example, the private-brand cereals sold by the co-ops and large chains usually cost 10 to 40 percent less than the equivalent advertised brands. Buy the simplest form without added sweetening or other ingredients, and even without shaping. (For example, co-op wheat shreds are only 25-30 cents a pound; shaped shredded wheat is almost twice as much.) Even dry cereals, of course, still do have useful nutritional value if they do not have large amounts of added sugar.

—Or you can use wheat germ, either by adding it to other cereals or by itself, at a relatively low price for the relatively high protein and other nutrients. Another type of dry cereal is Familia, a blend of several cereals, with some bran, wheat-germ substances, dried fruit and crushed almonds.

—If you feel you need vitamin fortification, and prefer to get it by eating cereal rather than by swallowing an inexpensive capsule (even this you may not need), Life is the least expensive of this type of cereal and yet has more protein and other nutrients than some of the others, as the table shows. The additional protein provided by some of the fortified cereals, even though from cereal rather than the more complete animal-source foods, is a nutritional advantage at, in some cases, not too high additional cost.

The Super-Convenience Hot Cereals

Even hot cereals now are being manufactured into fancier versions with added ingredients.

Oatmeal, particularly, that last stronghold of low-cost cereals and standby of large families, now has gone the way of dry cereals. Many new versions now on the market are presweetened and contain bits of apple, raisins, maple flavor and other ingredients. You now even can buy "quick" oatmeal, "instant" oatmeal and what can be described only as "instant instant" oatmeal.

The preflavored, super-convenience hot cereals show the fallacy of "convenience." The extra price you pay for the half minute you save by using the new "instant instant" oatmeal adds up to $4.30 an hour. In comparison, the typical average salary is $3 an hour. I sometimes think the average worker could make more money staying home and stirring oatmeal for his wife, sprinkling sugar on his kids' cornflakes and watering the fruit juice.

As the table of comparative costs of hot cereals shows, the addition of a few inexpensive ingredients and flavoring can quadruple the cost of your cereal—raising the price from as little as 1.2 cents an ounce to as much as 4.8 cents. Some of the extra ingredients featured in the names are even almost illusory. Oatmeal with Apples and Cinnamon, or Raisins and Spice, actually contains more added sugar than apples, raisins or spice, as the ingredients lists prove. The added "apples" consist of the tiniest chips of dehydrated apples you ever saw.

The real fallacy, from your point of view, is that you are paying at the rate of 77 cents a pound for the added sugar.

It is wise now to look at the weights and prices of hot cereals before you grab them off the shelf. Of three packages which seem to be the same size, one may provide 8 ounces, another 10, a third 12, at prices ranging from 33 to 43 cents, and costs per serving from 3.3 to 5.4 cents.

The table of comparative costs shows the savings available, not only from buying the simplest versions of hot cereal, but also the larger sizes. There also are some revealing differences shown in the costs of different brands.

The difference in cost per serving between some of the flavored hot cereals and the plain version is even greater than the comparative costs per ounce shown in the table. You need 1 ½ ounces of the flavored kind for a serving, compared with an ounce of the plain. Thus, the cost per serving of some flavored oatmeals comes to 6 cents, compared with 2.8 cents for plain instant oats, and 1.5 cents for quick oats.

The table of comparative costs shows that breakfast food values have little relation to price. Evaluating these foods on the basis of the protein—one of the costliest nutrients—provided, there are some sharp differences which can mean as much as $200 a year to a family of four.

For example, comparing costs of 20 grams of protein, which is a moderate amount that a family of four might expect this part of its breakfast to supply, here are the best values, with the cost of the 20 grams shown in cents in the parentheses:

Plain oatmeal (7.5 cents); muffins, made at home from a mix (7.5 cents); wheat germ (9.4 cents); farina (11 cents); bread or toast (14 cents); eggs (15 cents); pancakes (17 cents); 40 percent bran flakes (19.5 cents).

Here are the worst values in terms of 20 grams of protein:

Puffed wheat (33 cents); oatmeal with added sugar, apple bits and cinnamon (45 cents); puffed oats with sugar (46 cents); rice flakes (50 cents); puffed wheat with sugar and honey (56 cents); puffed rice (72 cents).

Notice how the higher price and reduced nutritive value of the sweetened and flavored hot cereals geometrically increases the cost of the protein in oatmeal actually 900 percent. Other poor values in this respect are the puffed dry cereals. You can get more nourishment for less money than puffed rice's real cost by serving steak for breakfast.

In the fortified cereals, for 20 grams of protein the lowest costs are: Life (14.8 cents); Fortified Oat Flakes (16.8 cents); Special K (17.5 cents). The most expensive for which protein data are available is Team (26.7 cents). These data are not provided in the labeling for King Vitaman and Kaboom, an omission that is a matter for concern. Since these products have added sugar (especially Kaboom), the protein value may be relatively low, as is usually the situation in presweetened cereals.

Don't be concerned that the cereal manufacturers will be angry, no matter what I say. As well as King Vitaman, Quaker Oats Co. makes Life, one of the relatively better values, and also a half dozen other good-value and poor-value cereals. So they can't lose. Nor can Kellogg's and the other big cereal manufacturers, all of whom compete with themselves with several brands.

But you can win.

COMPARATIVE FOOD VALUES PER SERVING
OF REPRESENTATIVE CEREALS
AND BREAKFAST FOODS*

	Cost per Serving**	Pro- tein	Cal- cium	Iron	Thia- mine	Ribo- flavin	Niacin
Plain Oatmeal	1.5¢	4.0	15.0	1.3	.17	.04	.28
Muffin (1.7 oz.)	1.5	4.0	74.0	.7	.08	.11	.7
Farina	1.7	3.2	7.1	.8	.1	.075	1.0
Bread, enriched (1 slice)	1.7	2.5	23.8	.7	.07	.06	.68
Pancakes (2) (1.1 oz.)	2.0	2.4	127.5	.9	.125	.095	.8
Corn Flakes, plain	2.4	2.2	4.8	.4	.12	.02	.58

	Cost per Serving**	Pro- tein	Cal- cium	Iron	Thia- mine	Ribo- flavin	Niacin
Bran Flakes, 40%	2.8¢	2.9	20.0	1.25	.1	.05	1.7
Cream of Rice	2.9	1.7	2.6	1.5	.12	.03	1.65
Shredded Wheat	3.0	2.8	12.2	.9	.06	.03	1.25
Wheat Flakes	3.3	2.9	11.6	1.25	.18	.04	1.4
Bran Flakes w/raisins	3.3	2.4	16.0	1.1	.09	.04	1.5
Oats, puffed	3.8	3.4	50.0	1.3	.28	.05	.5
Corn Flakes, sugar frosted	3.8	1.25	3.4	2.8	.12	.01	.5
Milk (½ cup)	4.0	4.8	146.0	.06	.04	.21	.09
Rice Flakes	4.2	1.7	8.2	.5	.1	.01	1.5
Oats, puffed w/sugar	4.4	1.9	20.0	1.25	.29	.03	.5
Egg (2 oz.)	5.0	6.5	27.25	1.2	5.25	.15	.025
Puffed Wheat w/sugar & honey	5.0	1.7	7.4	.94	.14	.05	1.8
Cream of Wheat (1.25 oz.) w/apples, cinnamon	5.6	2.2	n.a.	12.0	.15	.08	1.1
Puffed Rice	6.0	1.7	6.7	.5	.125	.01	1.25
Oatmeal (1.12 oz.) w/apples, cinnamon	6.1	2.7	n.a.	.7	.1	n.a.	n.a.
Puffed Wheat, plain	7.0	4.25	7.9	1.2	.16	.065	2.2

Fortified Cereals

	Cost per Serving**	Pro- tein	Cal- cium	Iron	Thia- mine	Ribo- flavin	Niacin
Life	3.8	5.1	75.0	1.5	1.0	1.2	10.0
Fortified Oat Flakes	4.3	5.1	43.0	20.0	.33	.40	3.33
Total	4.6	2.5	n.a.	10.0	1.0	1.2	10.0
Team	4.6	1.7	n.a.	1.5	.15	n.a.	2.0
Product 19	4.8	2.4	75.0	10.0	1.0	1.2	10.0
Special K	5.0	5.7	n.a.	3.3	.33	.39	3.3
King Vitaman	5.9	n.a.	n.a.	10.0	1.0	1.2	10.0
Kaboom	6.1	n.a.	n.a.	10.0	1.0	1.2	10.0
Wheat Germ	4.1	8.9	n.a.	2.5	.5	.22	1.4
Wheat Germ w/sugar'n honey	4.7	6.7	n.a.	1.8	.37	.16	1.0

*Protein value is expressed in grams; other nutrients, in milligrams.
**Serving is approximately 1 ounce as purchased except for egg (2 ounces); muffin (1.7 ounces); milk (4 ounces) and others as indicated in list.
n.a.: data not available.

COMPARATIVE COSTS OF HOT CEREALS*
(In order of ascending cost per serving)

	Pkg. Price	Net Contents	Cost per Oz.	Amt. for Serving	Cost per Serving
Oatmeals					
Quick Quaker Oats	63¢	42 oz.	1.6¢	1 oz.	1.5¢
Quick Quaker Oats	35	18	1.9	1	1.9
Quick H-O Oats	59	32	1.8	1-1/5	2.2
Quick H-O Oats	37	16	2.3	1-1/5	2.8
Instant H-O Oatmeal	37	16	2.3	1-1/5	2.8
Maypo Hot Oat Cereal	47	19	2.5	1-1/2	3.7
Instant H-O Oatmeal (8 packets)	41	10-2/3	3.9	1-1/3	4.1
Instant Quaker Oatmeal (10 packets)	49	10	4.9	1	4.9
Instant H-O Oatmeal w/raisins, spice (8 packets)	45	12	3.75	1-1/2	5.6
Instant Quaker Oatmeal w/apple, cinnamon (8 packets)	49	9	5.4	1-1/8	6.1
Instant Quaker Oatmeal w/dates, brown sugar (8 packets)	49	11	4.5	1-3/8	6.1
Instant Quaker Oatmeal w/raisins, spice (8 packets)	49	12	4.1	1-1/2	6.1
Maypo make-in-the-bowl maple oatmeal (8 packets)	49	9	5.4	1-1/8	6.1
Maypo make-in-the-bowl w/raisins, cinnamon (8 packets)	49	12	4.1	1-1/2	6.1
Instant Quaker Oatmeal w/maple, brown sugar (8 packets)	53	13	3.3	1-5/8	6.6
Other Cereals					
Pillsbury Farina	43	27-1/2	1.6	7/10	1.1
H-O Cream Farina	49	28	1.75	4/5	1.4
Nabisco Cream of Wheat	49	28	1.75	1	1.75
H-O Cream Farina	31	14	2.2	4/5	1.8
Instant Hot Ralston	37	18	2.0	1	2.0
Nabisco Cream of Wheat	34	14	2.4	1	2.4
Cream of Rice	47	16	2.9	1	2.9
Wheatena	49	22	2.2	1-1/2	3.3

	Pkg. Price	Net Contents	Cost per Oz.	Amt. for Serving	Cost per Serving
Other Cereals (Cont.)					
Instant Hot Ralston					
(10 packets)	43¢	10 oz.	4.3¢	1 oz.	4.3¢
Maltex Hot Cereal	49	20	2.45	1-3/4	4.3
Nabisco Mix'n Eat Cream of					
Wheat (10 packets)	45	10	4.5	1	4.5
Nabisco Mix'n Eat Cream of					
Wheat w/baked apples,					
cinnamon (8 packets)	45	10	4.5	1-1/4	5.6
Nabisco Mix'n Eat Cream of					
Wheat w/maple, brown					
sugar (8 packets)	45	10	4.5	1-1/4	5.6

*Price may vary among different cities and stores.

6

HOW GOVERNMENT PROGRAMS BOOST PRICES, ESPECIALLY OF MILK

Your food could cost a little less if the government stopped supporting farm prices by buying up so-called "surplus" commodities to help the farmers.

The commodity-purchase and other government price-support programs especially hurt moderate-income families in relation to the price of milk. A family with two children that hopes to use the nutritionally recommended 21 quarts a week finds its milk bill alone is in the neighborhood of $7 a week.

It is impossible, of course, to pay this much out of a total food budget of about $40 a week that a family of this size might spend for a moderate-cost food plan. In fact, $40 a week for food itself is impossible for the average worker earning, in 1971, $130 a week.

Some farmers certainly do need financial assistance. But the government spends $3 billion a year on buying commodities, and the public then pays additional untold billions in the form of higher prices, Meyer Parodneck, President of the Consumer-Farmer Milk Cooperative, points out.

The government also pays farmers, including corporations who own farms, to limit production of certain crops that are considered to be in "heavy" supply. These include rice, wheat and feed grains. The objective is to avoid "surpluses." But as noted in Chapter 1, retail food prices have risen more sharply in the late 1960's than most other commodities you have to buy. Thus, for these crop-control programs, whether mandatory or voluntary on the part of the farmers, as some are, you pay double: in taxes, and in higher food prices.

Instead of buying up commodities to keep up prices, direct subsidies would cost the government only about half as much, Parodneck, a long-time co-op milk distributor, points out. The government would save the extra costs paid for handling the "surplus" commodities to brokers, warehouses, processors and others in the daisy chain of food distribution. Much of the money the government spends to supposedly help the farmers goes to these people. (You would save too as retail prices found their own level.)

One of the most scandalous programs involves the price support of butter. This costly program "not only encourages the production of a product consumers do not want but makes those who do want it pay double its value," Parodneck charges.

The government's support of the price of butter is one of the reasons why the price of milk is high. "But when the consumer seeks to escape this trap by buying 'filled milk' (milk from which the butterfat has been extracted and vegetable fat substituted) the Agriculture Department then classifies this product as Class I milk, carrying the same price as fluid milk," Parodneck points out.

Some of the butter bought up and stored to keep up the price of milk even has been wasted because it turned rancid.

Another way that the price of milk you buy is forced up is through the double-price system used in the U.S. Agriculture Department milk-marketing orders. These orders regulate the price the farmer receives. Milk sold for use as drinking milk, called Class I milk, is sold at a higher price than Class II milk, sold to processors for manufacturing into dairy products such as cheese, ice cream and butter.

The theory behind this double-price system is that the milk for manufacturing purposes is "surplus" or leftover milk. For example, early in 1970, farmers were paid 15 cents a quart for milk to be sold as fluid milk, but only 10 cents for "manufacturing" milk, even though they are basically the same milk. (Somewhat lower standards of bacteria content and handling are permitted in some states for milk used for manufacturing but 70 percent of it, by USDA estimate, even now satisfies the fluid-milk standard.)

The use of such marketing orders to determine prices farmers in a marketing area receive and milk dealers and manufacturers pay, is said by the USDA to provide equal sharing of the value of their milk, no matter how it is used. The system provides equality, all right. All the farmers in the area are treated equally badly.

Ironically, when the high price of "drinking" milk forces families to reduce their use of it, the dairy-products manufacturers benefit, since there then is more "surplus" milk they can buy at the low Class II price. But both farmers and consumers are hurt—the farmer because the average price he gets for his milk is reduced proportionately when more of the milk goes into manufacturing.

Consumers are rarely represented at the hearings which set prices for milk under the marketing orders. The hearings may be held in remote places and usually consumer organizations are not notified of them. Consumer organizations, ill-financed and undermanned as they are, often would not have the available experts to present the consumer point of view and debate the technical data, even if they were notified of the hearings.

The way milk is priced is obsolete and cost-raising in another way. The 1969 White House Conference on Food, Nutrition and Health recommended that milk be priced on the basis of its nonfat solids rather than on its butterfat content as now.

But also, milk prices need to be reduced by eliminating barriers such as artificial local "sanitary" and other regulations such as barn construction (really aimed at favoring local dairy interests) impeding the flow of milk from Midwest dairy states to large population centers, and also through economies in retail distribution, encouragement of competition and active surveillance and prosecution of local milk price-fixing, and through encouragement of low-cost milk stations such as those sponsored by the Consumer-Farmer Milk Co-op in New York.

Farmers get very angry at any suggestion that the price of milk is higher than it need be, or that butter is not universally wanted anymore, or not a good value, or even not necessarily healthy for some people. When I wrote in my syndicated column in 1967 the simple fact that margarine has the same food value as butter at one-third the cost, the newspapers published in Wisconsin and surrounding states by the Midland Cooperatives discontinued the column after seventeen years of publishing it. They had received many complaints, even cancellations of feed orders, from farmer-members and customers.

Much more seriously, the National Dairy Council has attacked the American Heart Association for its recommendations for reduced use of saturated fat as in butter and whole milk in order to reduce cholesterol levels. The Heart Association reports that dairy interests even have warned that they will not contribute to the Heart Fund.

As well as the dual-price marketing order system, another problem that has plagued consumers from time to time is local price-fixing. Sometimes this is done officially by states, either by establishing the retail price or, almost as effectively, by limiting the number of licenses issued to dealers. Occasionally state authorities even have limited the number of outlets or the territories or dealers the distributor could service. Such tactics, claimed to be aimed at preventing price wars, also freeze out new competitors and prevent price reductions.

But sometimes the price also is fixed unofficially by distributors, who at times even have tried to stop such cost-cutting innovations as gallon jugs, milk depots and vending machines. For example, for eighteen years Denver prohibited the sale of milk in gallon jugs. When gallon jugs were finally allowed, the price of milk in half-gallon containers came down to meet the competition, the U.S. Agriculture Department reported.[10]

In Louisville, too, the distribution of milk in gallon jugs at a lower price ended a long-standing unfair differential of 1 cent for homogenized milk over the price of cream-line. It costs the dairies virtually nothing to homogenize milk. It merely passes through a machine which shakes it to distribute the butterfat evenly. You could do that with your bare hands by shaking the bottle briskly.

Often price-fixing by local distributors is unofficial, with no formal meetings or written agreements. The distributors usually will follow the price lead of the largest distributor. Without genuine competition in the prices charged consumers, distributors tend to compete for retailer preference through gifts, loans and special services—which further adds to distribution costs.

Price-fixing is especially unfair to moderate-income consumers and lower-price minimum-service stores which could and would sell milk for less.

Sometimes the authorities catch up. In 1967 a New York County grand jury indicted twelve milk companies and a number of individuals for conspiracy to fix prices. Official investigations and similar charges have occurred in other cities from time to time.

Local price-fixing by distributors is often designed to protect home delivery by maintaining a narrow differential between store and home prices. My own study of Bureau of Labor Statistics data shows that in various cities the difference may range from nothing at all or only a cent to as much as 8 cents a quart, with the national average difference about 4 cents. It is interesting to see that in Atlanta, where there is virtually no difference in price between stores and home delivery, the store price is the highest of any large city in the country (4 cents higher than national average), although Atlanta otherwise is not a high-cost city for food.

Similarly, in Kansas City, where the differential is only 1 cent, the price of milk in stores is higher than in St. Louis, where the differential is 4 cents.

Distributive costs are the real problem. While the farmer in 1970 got a nickel a quart more than he did in 1955, you were paying a dime more. From 1964 to 1968, average milk prices received by farmers rose 27 percent; average retail prices rose 32 percent.

What can you do to protect yourself from the high price, especially if you live in one of the higher-cost milk cities? It is noticeable that even in the same region milk costs a lot more in some towns than in others nearby; for example, only 30 cents in Pittsburgh and Baltimore, compared with 33 cents in Philadelphia and Atlanta.

For one thing, don't try to boycott milk, as has been suggested occasionally. If not as reasonable as it could be, it still is a reasonable food compared with many others. A quart of milk is 2.2 pounds. So figure it costs you 13-14 cents a pound. Milk still costs no more than the heavily used carbonated beverages, which provide no nutrition at all other than sugar.

If you can't afford to buy all the fluid milk your family needs, then use nonfat milk powder to make reconstituted milk at 12 cents a quart (or as little as 8 cents in bulk sizes) and mix this with fresh milk. You also can use the nonfat milk powder in cooking and baking to add extra nutrition to desserts, cakes, soups, meat patties and loaves, etc.

The price-support activities of the Agriculture Department include buying nonfat dry milk and storing it in warehouses, with a resultant increase in the price you must pay for this product too. The increasing popularity of diet drinks also has helped raise the price of nonfat dry milk. Still, if not as reasonable as it once was, it still is cheap enough to actually be the No. 1 food value in the country in terms of the nutrients provided for the price. A quart of reconstituted nonfat milk gives you 36 grams of protein at a cost of 12 cents, compared with 65 cents for the same amount of protein from round steak and even from hamburger, 33 cents.

As well as the protein, nonfat dry milk provides all the minerals, lactose and water-soluble vitamins of whole milk—in fact, everything but the butterfat. The vitamin A missing with the butterfat can be supplied by green and yellow vegetables, margarine or liver in a meal.

Another cost cutter is evaporated milk for cooking. It does have the butterfat, but costs less than fresh milk.

Powdered whole milk is another potential money-saver, but until now has not been popular because the delicate fresh milk flavor was lost in the drying process. The USDA has developed a spray-dried whole milk which it believes has comparable taste quality to fresh milk on the basis of pilot taste tests made in the late 1960's. When available in stores, the estimated saving would be about 15 percent. "Concentrated milk" also is becoming available in more stores at similar savings. It is a concentrated fluid which you mix with two parts water.

Butter in recent years has cost three times as much as margarine. Margarine fortified with vitamin A has as much food value as butter, and does not turn rancid so quickly. In fact, some months of the year butter provides only 6,000 units of vitamin A per pound, but margarine always has 15,000 units.

Private-brand milk sold by large retailers has been a help to consumers. It usually sells for a penny a quart less, and it is hard for processors to differentiate private brands from advertised brands in the case of milk because both must meet specific standards. Milk is milk and there is no way the processors can claim that an advertised brand of the same grade is any better.

But they can try to differentiate with a minor change in ingredients, as they did in California in 1966. Home economist Mary Gullberg reported in *Co-op News* that a distributor advertised its milk as "5 percent richer than minimum state standards." The minimum standard was 3.5 percent butterfat and 9 percent nonfat solids, which meant merely that the claimed richer milk has a nutritionally insignificant 3.7 percent butterfat and 9 percent solids. The milk did not really meet the state definition of 4.2 percent butterfat for "extra rich" milk.

A higher price for "enriched" milk with added vitamin D is definitely not in your interest. A Public Health Service official, Dr. Arnold Schaefer, testified before Congress that it costs less than a penny per hundred gallons to thus "enrich" milk.

"Diet" and Other High-Price Milks

As though the price of milk were not high enough, processors have found ways to charge even more, through various diet and other special milks and yogurt.

A product sold as "Fortified Diet Milk," for example, is merely skim milk with some added nonfat milk and a little whole milk. It has 1 percent butterfat. Yet diet milks such as this one and Light n' Lively sell for as much as whole milk: 29 to 32 cents a quart. You can mix a similar "diet milk" with about three cups of reconstituted nonfat milk and one of ordinary milk, adding an extra tablespoon or two of nonfat milk powder and your own flavorings, at a cost of approximately 18 cents.

Peculiarly, Fortified Diet Milk is advertised as "99 percent fat free." Technically, that is accurate. But with that reasoning, even the usual 3.5 percent whole milk is 96.5 percent fat free.

The advertising for some "instant breakfasts" has been

criticized for its nutritional claims. In 1970 the Carnation Co. agreed to discontinue what the Federal Trade Commission called unwarranted claims that Carnation Instant Breakfast had the nutritional value of two eggs, bacon, toast and orange juice. The FTC had complained that Carnation failed to reveal that some of the claimed nutrients were provided by the additional milk you mix with the product.

In actual fact, such instant breakfasts are basically nonfat dry milk plus sugar (called sucrose on the label), flavorings, fillers to provide bulk and added synthetic vitamins. If you calculate the cost per pound of such fractionally-sized packages as 65 to 69 cents for 7½ ounces, the real cost is approximately $1.50 a pound, compared with about 55 cents for the basic skim milk.

Many of the flavored and chocolate milk drinks for children and ingredients sold to mix into their milk can double and even triple the cost of milk. Frosted Shakes, a powder advertised as containing "dry ice cream mix," actually has as its leading ingredients sugar and vegetable oils. If you figure out the real cost, it's a dollar a pound.

Great Shakes, a chocolate-flavored mix, which you mix with milk, has as its leading ingredient sugar, followed by malted milk, cocoa and various thickeners and flavorings.

You also can buy already prepared milkshakes for your kids. At 18 cents for 10 ounces, this comes to 58 cents a quart for milk with added sugar, thickeners and artificial flavor.

Canned chocolate drinks charge a whole-milk price for a product that is, in order of importance, water, nonfat milk, sugar, cocoa and the usual chemicals. If you buy premixed "quick" cocoa you pay a high cocoa price for cheaper ingredients such as nonfat milk and sugar.

Frances Cerra, enterprising consumer reporter for *Newsday* (Long Island, New York), found that the price of even premixed cocoa jumped another 33 percent when packed in individual packets. That is a high price to pay to save ladling out two teaspoons of cocoa, Miss Cerra commented.

Imitation and Synthetic Milks

"Filled" milks had a brief popularity in some states during the late 1960's, but more recently have become less available.

"Filled" milk, also called imitation milk or mellorine, is different from synthetic milk. The filled milk, even though (in most areas) it is labeled imitation milk, has a base of milk solids but a vegetable oil is substituted for the milk fat. This substitution reduces the cost to the consumer about 3 to 5 cents a quart.

Often, however, the substitute vegetable oil used is coconut oil, since its flavor and properties make it a palatable substitute for butterfat, government home economists note. But coconut oil, unlike most vegetable oil, is highly saturated and thus perhaps undesirable for mature people on low-cholesterol diets.

Otherwise, the nutritive values of filled milk are like those of milk.

Imitation milk made with coconut oil also has been criticized as undesirable for infants' formula, since it lacks an essential fatty acid.

In contrast, synthetic milk, also called imitation milk in some areas, contains no milk materials, but substitutes a soybean derivative that has less protein than milk and may or may not have the important vitamins and minerals of milk added.

The Water in Your Cheese

As meat has become more expensive, so has cheese. The sharp rise in the price has even less justification, and little relation to the much smaller increase in the price of the milk from which it is made. From 1965 to 1970 the price of American process cheese, one of the less costly and most widely sold varieties, rose from 75 cents a pound to 95 cents to $1; a rise of 33 percent, compared with 20 percent for milk.

Moreover, cheese increasingly is manufactured into processed and blended types with additional water so it is easier to spread, and added water-retaining ingredients such as bits of olive, pimento, vegetables and vegetable gum. It is then subjected to more expensive packaging, such as single-wrapping and jars.

Thus the cost is raised additionally while the food value frequently is reduced.

As the table in this chapter shows, various varieties and processed cheeses may have anywhere from 32 to 60 percent water, often euphemistically called on the labels "moisture."

The chart also shows that you get the most protein for your money in natural cheddar, not in the packaged processed cheeses. And protein is the expensive nutrient—especially protein from animal sources, as cheese has.

Cottage cheese, even with its high moisture content, is the best value in terms of protein cost—actually about only one-fifth the cost of the protein in cream cheese. Even Neufchâtel is much less costly in any terms than the similar cream cheese. Note also that you pay 25 percent more for a staple cheese such as American if you buy it presliced. Cheese sold cubed or grated also costs significantly more than wedges or sticks.

In shopping for cheese, especially note the differences between "pasteurized process" cheese, "cheese food," "cheese spread" and "imitation process cheese spread." While the basic cheddar and Swiss cheese from which these processed varieties are made cannot by definition have more than 39 and 41 percent water respectively, cheese "food" may have as much as 43 percent, cheese "spread" as much as 59 percent, and "imitation cheese spread" even more. (The brand we checked had 54 percent.)

Many of the jarred spreading cheeses have 52 to 60 percent water. Not only do they thus have a correspondingly reduced protein value, but a true cost per pound of $1.20 to $1.30 when you break down the price of the various 3½-, 4- and 5-ounce jars. Neufchâtel in bulk is 68 cents a pound; in jars, it comes out to $1.25.

As with other processed foods, processed cheeses have their ingredients listed on the label in order of importance.

What happens to cheese on the way to the factory, and then to your table, is a revealing lesson in modern economics and how to buy your money's worth.

The Agricultural Marketing Service traced the path of this cheese from the day the farmers delivered the raw milk to three cheese factories, to the day you stopped at a cheese counter and bought a package of it. These facts and figures show how small the labor cost is in manufacturing and retailing such items, and the exaggerated prices manufacturers charge the public for "convenience" foods.

The prices mentioned are higher now, since this study was made in the late 1950's, but the relationships are approximately the same.

The raw milk delivered by the farmers cost the cheese factories 28.2 cents for the quantity equivalent to one pound of processed cheese. It cost just 4.2 cents a pound to manufacture this milk into cheese, including all labor, equipment and overhead costs. The factories also had to add a small amount for boxes and hauling.

The cheese factories in turn sold the cheese to assemblers for an average price of 31.7 cents.

The assemblers graded and paraffined the big wheels of cheese and resold it to processors for an average price of 32.3 cents a pound.

So far, nobody had made much money on this cheese. But now the processors have the cheese. These are the big companies who change the form of the original cheddar slightly and package it under brand names.

The processors ground the cheese into small granules, blended it with other cheeses, added coloring, salt, emulsifier and water, and cooked it for five minutes, then machine-packaged the melted cheese.

The first fact to notice is that the processors added approximately 7 percent water to the natural cheddar. When you buy a pound of this cheese, you get 14.9 ounces of the original cheese and 1.1 ounces of water.

The processor then took his softened, watered cheese and sold two lots of it to retailers and jobbers at 37 and 37.8 cents, and one lot at a much higher price of 47.3 cents. The two cheaper lots were sold as 2-pound and 5-pound loaves. But the higher-priced lot had been sliced and packaged in half-pound packages. For this, the processor actually got 10 cents more a pound, or more than twice as much as the entire cost of manufacturing the original cheese.

A chain store that bought the high-priced sliced cheese paid the transportation charges, marked up the price 31 percent and sold the cheese to you for 62 cents a pound. The 2-pound loaves were bought by supermarkets, which charged 47.5 to 49.5 cents a pound, and by the chain store, which charged 52.5 cents. The 5-pound loaves were sold to small grocery and delicatessen stores. They charged 49 to 75 cents per pound, cut from the loaf.

Here's what we can learn from this incident:

1. The more the manufacturers process foods, the more they

charge, and often out of proportion to the value added. It only costs 4 cents a pound to manufacture the original cheese, but to soften it and form it into loaves adds another 6 cents. If the processor also slices it and wraps it in half-pound packages, he charges you another full dime.

This is called "built-in maid service" and is used to justify the high prices charged for "convenience" foods.

Moreover, by buying processed cheese, which is easier to spread, instead of natural cheddar, the consumer paid 4½ cents for a little over 1 ounce of water.

2. For the same cheese, some people paid as little as 47½ cents a pound, and some as much as 75 cents, depending on where they bought it, and in what size package and under what brand name.

3. Actual labor costs of manufacturing and retailing the cheese were only a fraction of the price charged. The entire basic manufacturing cost of the original cheese, including labor, machinery and other overhead, was only 4 cents a pound.

You can glean useful buying tips from the chart of cheese costs:

—Of two brands of American-type cheese spread (primarily American cheese with added water) selling at the same price, one may have only 46 percent water, the other 50 percent.

—Imitation cheese spreads such as Chef's Delight have a high water content. But at a low price of under 40 cents a pound, they appear to be a reasonable protein value because of the low butterfat content (only 5 percent) and the high proportion of nonfat milk used in their manufacture.

—The addition of water to natural cheeses reduces their food value without always a corresponding reduction in price. A noticeable example found by Mrs. Jessen in comparing ingredients was Wispride cheese "spread" with 52 percent moisture at 6 ounces for 51 cents ($1.36 a pound). But the same brand of cold pack cheese sold in wedges with only 44 percent moisture was 8 ounces for 57 cents ($1.14 a pound). This also is an example of how selling products in different-sized packages makes comparing values difficult for the consumer.

—Neufchâtel bought as such is a moderate-cost soft cheese

and higher in protein value than the similarly priced cream cheese. But with the addition of flavoring such as pimento or bits of clam, or blended with a smaller amount of blue cheese, and sold in small packages, as party snacks, the price jumps 47 percent. Similarly, whipped cream cheese, which merely has air added, costs 50 percent more. The appearance of size can be a fooler.

—While American cheese in loaf or bulk style is the best protein value on the list except for cottage cheese, note how the price jumps if the cheese is sliced, and jumps again if the slices are wrapped.

The Ice Cream Problem

Many complaints are made about modern ice cream, especially the amount of over-run (additional air) in the cheaper brands, differences in quality and confusion over different types.

A major problem is that ice cream is sold by volume rather than weight. In our own survey, we weighed different brands sold at different prices and found, for example, that three different brands of half-gallon containers sold by the same supermarket weighed 39, 44 and 45 ounces. But the price range was even greater—75 cents, $1.03 and $1.29 a half-gallon.

Thus the cheapest ice cream, despite the fact that it had more air and weighed 5 and 6 ounces less than the others, still cost the least per pound of solids: 31 cents, as against 37 cents for the medium-priced brand and 46 cents for the costliest (French type). However, the cheaper brands also often have more water.

For protection against excessive adulteration, government standards restrict the addition of air and water to the ice cream mix. Ice cream is required to weigh at least 4½ pounds (72 ounces) per gallon, or 36 ounces to the half-gallon. The low-priced supermarket private brands we checked were above this limit. However, it was not possible to determine the differences in water content and actual solids. The minimum standards, which are quite low, merely specify that the solids may not be less than 1.6 pounds (22 ounces) per gallon. Thus a half-gallon or 32-ounce container of ice cream may have as much as 21 ounces of water (by weight).

All products labeled "ice cream" also must meet minimum government standards for ingredients. They must contain at least 20 percent by weight of milk solids, of which at least 10 percent must be milk fat. French ice cream and frozen custard also must have a specified amount of egg yolk solids.

"Ice milk" must have not less than 11 percent of total milk solids, of which not less than 2 percent and not more than 7 percent are milk fat.

"Fruit sherbets" must have not less than 1 percent total milk solids, but not more than 5 percent total milk solids content, of which not less than 1 percent but not more than 2 percent are milk fat.

MOISTURE LIMITS OF CHEESE VARIETIES*

Parmesan	32%
Romano	34
Cheddar	39
Gruyère	39
Cold pack or club cheese, various types	39-42
Swiss	41
Gorgonzola	42
Pasteurized processed cheese, various types	40-44
Monterey	44
Brick	44
Pasteurized processed cheese food	44
Provolone	45
Edam	45

Blue	46
Muenster	46
Cream cheese	55
Pasteurized processed cheese spread	44-60
Neufchâtel	65
Cottage cheese	80

*The figure listed indicates that the cheese must have less than this amount of moisture (a euphemism for water).

TYPICAL COSTS OF VARIOUS CHEESES

	Price per Lb.	Maximum Moisture	Gms. Protein per Lb.	Cost of 100 Gms. Protein
Cottage cheese	39¢	80%	61.7 gms.	63¢
American, bulk	82	43	105.2	79
sliced	$1.04	43	105.2	99
wrapped slices	$1.30	43	105.2	$1.24
Process "spread," American				
loaf	72	46-50	*	*
5 oz. jar	$1.36	50	*	*
spray can	$1.26	50	*	*
Cheddar, natural mild	95	39	113.4	84
"food," wedge	$1.08	44	89.8	$1.20
"spread," container	$1.36	52	*	*
Swiss, domestic, bulk	$1.19	32	124.7	96
wrapped slices	$1.30	32	124.7	$1.04
Muenster, bulk	99	46	n.a.	n.a.
sliced	$1.21	46	n.a.	n.a.
Imitation cheese "spread"	38	62	**	**
Cheez Whiz, blend of American, brick, muenster	98	52	**	**

	Price per Lb.	Maximum Moisture	Gms. Protein per Lb.	Cost of 100 Gms. Protein
Neufchâtel, plain	68¢	65%	42.6 gms.	$1.36
flavored "spreads"	$1.16	65	42.6	$2.72
Cream cheese, natural	68	55	36.3	$1.87
whipped	$1.03	55	36.3	$2.84
Parmesan, grated	$1.78	32	163.3	$1.09
Blue cheese	$1.33	46	97.5	$1.36

*No close estimate of protein value was feasible because of variations in water and butterfat in different brands. If an approximate protein value of 75 grams per pound is assumed as typical for "cheese spreads," then loaf-style spreads with about 50 per cent water and 20 per cent fat would have a cost of about 95 cents for 100 grams of protein: not unreasonable but not quite as good protein value as standard American loaf or bulk cheese or cheddar. But the process cheese spreads in jars, containers and spray cans would be inordinately costly for the protein value.

**While no data are available on protein value, imitation cheeses may be high in protein despite high water content because of nonfat milk ingredients and resultant low butterfat.

n.a.: data not available

CHAPTER

7

INVENTED BREAKFAST "DRINKS" AND THE FACTS ABOUT VITAMIN C

Of all the modern "foods" technologists have invented, the heavily advertised imitation "breakfast drinks" and sugar-water beverages are among the most widespread and potentially deceptive money wasters.

There are two types of such beverages. One is the canned "drinks," "ades" and "punches" usually sold in big 46-ounce cans. The other is the imitation "orange juice" concentrates and "instant breakfast drinks" in dry form.

If you read the labels of the canned drinks, you will see that the leading ingredients are sugar and water. For example, obscurely enough on the side of the can, Welch's Orange Drink lists as its ingredients "water, sugar, orange juice concentrate, citric acid, cellulose gum, vegetable oil and gum, vitamin C, artificial color, orange oil."

The other "drinks" list similar ingredients, led by water and sugar. But none of the labels tell you *what percentage water and what percentage orange juice.* As far back as 1964 the Food and Drug Administration announced it was considering establishing standards of identity for various types of diluted juices and beverages. Under these proposals the various beverages would be required to state the actual amount of real fruit juice—for example, "50 percent fruit juice drink, pineapple-grapefruit," "30 percent fruit juice grapeade" and "10 percent fruit juice orange drink."

By late 1970 these standards and the accompanying more informative labeling had not yet been effected, leaving the public still confused as to whether a canned or frozen beverage labeled "orange drink" has more or less orange juice than one labeled "orange ade," or even how much real juice two different brands of "orange drink" have.

One *approximate* guide to what these beverages provide is an unofficial model code adopted by the Association of Food and Drug Officials. It calls for at least 50 percent fruit juice in "juice drinks," 25 percent in "ades" except lemonade or limeade and 10 percent in "drinks or punch." Anything under 10 percent is supposed to be labeled a "flavored drink."

Thus, at best, the big cans of "drinks" are 90 percent water. But even this code is only a recommendation and has no legal force. Other trade sources and state agencies have reported that some of the canned drinks are as little as 6 percent real juice and even less. The manufacturers carefully guard these data on their own brands. In researching fruit "drinks" for this book, Mrs. Jessen received this letter from the "customer relations" department of the A&P: ". . . the percentage of water and sugar in our Orange Drink cannot be revealed as it is a formula secret. We can advise, however, that, based on the ingredient statement on the label, sugar is one of the major ingredients." That much we knew. We can read labels too. Only the consumer co-ops, to my knowledge, reveal the actual percentages: nectars, 40 percent real juice; pineapple-grapefruit drink, 50 percent juice; grape drink, 30 percent juice. When the industry dropped the grape juice content in grape drinks to 25 percent in the late 1960's, the co-ops maintained theirs at 30, Mary Gullberg, home economist for Berkeley, California, co-ops, reports.

The low juice content of such "drinks" has become both a financial and nutritional issue. As the chart of comparative costs in this chapter shows, from a money point of view the customary 4-ounce serving of real orange juice typically costs about 50 percent less than a 6-ounce serving of canned orange "drink." Further, since the real juice, ounce for ounce, provides about 70 percent more vitamin C, the cost of this nutrient in real juice is only about one-third to a half the cost of the same amount in the diluted drinks, without even counting the additional nutrients provided by the real juice such as vitamin A, calcium, some of the B vitamins and even a little protein.

Even with their added synthetic vitamin C, an ounce of the sugar-water "drinks" provides only 5 milligrams of vitamin C (ascorbic acid) compared with about 12.5 per ounce of orange juice, and about 11 for grapefruit juice.

This means that it takes 6 ounces of most orange "drinks" to provide the 30 milligrams of vitamin C considered to be the *minimum* daily requirement. You get this much in just 2½ ounces of orange juice at less than half the price of the "drinks." The usual 4-ounce serving of orange juice provides about 50 milligrams of vitamin C. This is nutritionally more desirable than the minimum 30, which really is a desirable minimum only for children.

The two-fold problem is that many moderate-income families tend to buy such "drinks" for use as breakfast drinks because they seem cheap, and thus deprive themselves nutritionally, and even if such drinks are used only as auxiliary beverages for children, they cost more than adding water and sugar to real juices.

While the FDA still was temporizing over requiring more informative labeling, the Federal Trade Commission in 1970 did act to cut down the nutritional claims for "orange drinks."

The FTC charged that the manufacturer of Hi-C, the Coca-Cola Co., made false nutritional claims, and asserted that the name "Hi-C" itself is misleading. In fact, the FTC charged, Hi-C is less nutritious, even though often more expensive, than real orange juice.

While the Coca-Cola Co. defended Hi-C with large ads asserting the product contributed "significant" amounts of vitamin C to daily needs, the FTC took particular exception to claims that the product has "lots of vitamin C" and was made with fresh fruit. It is not made with fresh fruit and has only one-half to one-third the vitamin C of orange juice, the government agency said. (Ads actually said, "You wanted a drink. . .that had to be naturally sweetened and made from fresh fruit. . . that had lots of vitamin C. . .so we gave you Hi-C." In actual fact, the list of ingredients shows no fresh fruit juice listed, and the sweetener is sugar, which could be interpreted as a "natural" sweetener.)

While the chart in this chapter shows Hawaiian Punch as weaker in vitamin C than other drinks, the manufacturer informed us that late in 1970 the vitamin C in its "Orange" and "Pineapple" drinks was increased to 88.7 milligrams per 6 ounces from the previous 30 milligrams per 8 ounces. The old stock in stores is expected to be completely replaced by the end of 1971.

The best buy for the nutrition you get is frozen orange juice, a better buy than not only the "drinks," but also better than the other real juices such as grapefruit, pineapple and tomato. (If not enriched, pineapple juice is relatively low in vitamin C.)

The Coca-Cola Co. still has its flank protected. If its advertising of Hi-C is restricted, it also makes two of the leading frozen orange juice concentrates.

The so-called "instant breakfast drinks" are also questionable. These are really invented foods consisting mainly of sugar, flavorings, artificial coloring and added vitamin C, with one or two other added vitamins, plus fillers (even vegetable oil). Revealingly, Start, Tang and Awake are all made by General Foods.

So you can't complain that there is no competition in the food business. Different divisions of General Foods compete against each other in advertising, invented product names, price and variations of the vitamins and flavorings they add to these synthetic beverages.

Start and Tang are powders. You add water. But Awake is the silliest idea of all. It is really a frozen concentrate of sugar syrup (water and sugar) with the added flavorings and synthetic vitamins. Presumably the merchandising strategy in making this a frozen concentrate instead of a powder, and putting it in the store's freezer cabinet, is so it can attract shoppers looking for frozen juice. Awake may benefit from sleepy shoppers in more ways than one.

General Foods' Awake also competes in the frozen concentrate department with General Foods' Orange Plus, another evasively advertised fluid. This is "a frozen concentrate for imitation orange juice," really half orange juice with sugar syrup, corn syrup, flavorings, colorings, thickeners such as vegetable oil and added vitamins. A 9-ounce can of Orange Plus is advertised as providing "as much beverage" as two 6-ounce cans of frozen orange juice—certainly, since the directions instruct you to add more water than for reconstituted real juice (four cans compared with three). You can make more "beverage" with anything by adding more water.

The synthetic drinks are even less expensive for their vitamin C than orange juice concentrate, but do not have all of the other nutrients of the real juice, although Orange Plus has some. Synthetic vitamin C is cheap. We figure that a 9-ounce jar of Tang for 59 cents gives you about 10 cents worth of vitamin C plus a penny's worth of vitamin A. Thus, you pay $1.05 a pound for a product that is mostly sugar with flavorings and 11 cents worth of vitamins. Sugar is 13 cents a pound.

The Soft Drink Mixes

The soft drink mixes such as Kool-Aid and Funny Face are basically merely flavorings with little nutritive value except sugar. The unsweetened versions of these mixes have as their leading ingredient synthetic fumaric acid, an additive on the FDA permitted list, which provides acidity and prevents caking. Here is a case in which an additive has become the basic food product. The sweetened versions do have a small amount of added vitamin C—1.25 milligrams per ounce. You would have to drink 24 ounces to get 30 milligrams. The seemingly cheap price is a fooler. You can make a more nourishing drink with the same vitamin C value by mixing nine parts of water with one or orange juice, and adding sugar, at about one-third the cost of Kool-Aid (also made by our old friend General Foods), and half that of the less expensive Funny Face.

The "Thirst Quenchers"

As many old-timers remember, water is a thirst quencher. Recently food manufacturers discovered that if they added sweetenings, salts, flavorings and in some cases minerals to water they could bottle it and sell it as rapid thirst quenchers under such names as Gatorade, Energade and Olympade. These are offered supposedly for athletes but all "active people" are urged, in repetitive TV advertising, to drink the stuff.

A 12-ounce can of a widely promoted "thirst quencher" —Energade—consists of 11 ounces of water plus 1 ½ ounces of sugar and dextrose (corn sugar) plus a blend of sodium and potassium salts. The "thirst quenchers" also have various flavorings and preservatives. The function of the salts is like that of a salt tablet—to replace body salts lost through perspiration.

Energade at least also has some unspecified percentage of concentrated orange juice. Some of the other "quenchers," such as Gatorade, have merely sugars, salts and citrus flavoring. The price for bottled or canned water with sugars, salts and flavoring is high—about 8 cents for an 8-ounce glass in bottles (about the same price as milk), and 12 in cans.

The General Foods version of the "thirst quenchers" is a dry mix called Instant Replay. The ingredients are so similar to the General Foods' Tang, it almost seems as though the company's food chemists had simply taken Tang, modified it a little, added salts and minerals and sold it as a "thirst quencher." Instant Replay actually is 90 percent sugar but this is supposed to be confidential information, so don't tell anyone else.

Instant Replay, while still expensive for what it provides, is a little cheaper, since the water is not shipped with it—6 cents for an 8-ounce glass. It also provides added vitamin C.

Other Sources of Vitamin C

While vitamin C is one of the nutrients most often found short in American diets, it really is unnecessary to be overly-influenced by promotions for high-cost diluted or synthetic beverages with added vitamin C. Not only do real juices offer a base for beverages at a lower cost, but there are many other sources of vitamin C in the ordinary foods you eat. Among these are cabbage, tomatoes, potatoes, many fruits and many green vegetables, especially the leafy green kind such as spinach, kale and collards, and also broccoli and brussels sprouts.

But vitamin C is the most fragile of vitamins. It is soluble in water and also can be destroyed by exposure to air; thus, it often is lost through careless or unknowing home-cooking methods and handling while in the stores.

The most dramatic example of the effects of such mishandling came to light in Canada some years ago. Medical investigators sought to find out why malnutrition was more widespread in Newfoundland than the rest of Canada, to the extent that the overall death rate was 20 percent greater.

Among other nutritional lacks, the medical teams found that the Islanders suffered from vitamin C deficiency. For one thing, the women habitually boiled their potatoes *after* peeling, cooking out much of the vitamin C. Too, they cooked them in the morning for the evening meal, so the rest of the vitamin C fled. They boiled their cabbage for one to two hours, robbing themselves of much of the vitamin C from that source.

Infants and older folks are most apt to be short of vitamin C, some nutritionists believe. The oldsters, especially elderly men living alone, frequently neglect to eat fruits. Middle-aged people, and especially women, tend to eat more fruits and vegetables. Nor is the lack of vitamin C as important in the middle years as in babies and seniors.

As the chart of "C-rich" fruits and vegetables shows, the more you cook, the less "C" you have left. Cabbage will give you 50 milligrams in only 100 grams (3 ½ ounces) of shredded raw cabbage (cole slaw). But cook it lengthily in a lot of water and you have left only 32 milligrams in a 170-gram cup of boiled cabbage. As noted earlier in this book, the fresh versions of foods prepared at home usually have more nutrition than highly processed versions. In the particular case of potatoes, reconstituted dehydrated potato granules have only about half the vitamin C of mashed potatoes made from raw potatoes.

Wild or cultivated rose fruits, called rose hips, are one of the richest sources of vitamin C. They make a jam with a flavor like raspberry, or a fruit beverage or puree. In Norway, rose hip powder is used in the fruit soups popular in that country, and is sprinkled on breakfast cereal.

With all these natural sources, and with knowledgeable kitchen care, it is hardly necessary to pay a high price for invented beverages and other products promoted as having added synthetic vitamin C. In fact, an unnecessarily high intake won't serve any useful purpose. The body can accumulate a pool of vitamin C, but an excess is excreted. (There remains, of course, the unresolved issue of whether massive intakes of vitamin C can help decrease colds, as argued by Linus Pauling and sensationalized by newspaper reports. Some medical authorities who have done research on vitamin C differ with Professor Pauling. But the fact that this controversy will not be settled for years until more studies can be made, did not stop many people from rushing to buy all the vitamin C they could find. In early 1971 retailers and wholesalers were out of stock for weeks because of the sudden demand. Adolph Kamil, Berkeley Co-op pharmacist, reported that the rush for vitamin C began even before Pauling's book on the subject was available in that area, so very few actually could have read it.)

COMPARATIVE COSTS OF BREAKFAST DRINKS AND VITAMIN C

	Usual Serving Costs	30 mgs. Vit. C Costs
	(4 oz.)	
Orange Juice, cans, bottles		
Private Brand, 46-oz. can	3.6¢	2.1¢
Private Brand, 32-oz. bottle	4.8	2.9
Tropicana, 32-oz. bottle	5.2	3.0
Orange Juice, frozen concentrate		
A & P, 6 oz.	2.8	1.8
Bohack,* 6 oz.	3.2	1.9
Libby, 6 oz.	3.6	2.2
Minute Maid, 6 oz.	4.0	2.4
Snow Crop, 6 oz.	4.4	2.7
Pathmark,* 12 oz.	2.6	1.6
A & P, 12 oz.	2.7	1.6
Snow Crop, 12 oz.	3.6	2.2
Orange Plus (imitation orange juice)	4.0	1.6
Grapefruit Juice		
Private Brand, 6 oz., concentrate	4.0	2.8
Private Brand, 46-oz. can	4.4	3.1

	Usual Serving Costs	30 mgs. Vit. C Costs
Pineapple Juice, (vit. C enriched)**		
Pathmark, 46-oz. can	2.4¢	2.4¢
A & P, 46-oz. can	2.6	2.6
Dole, 46-oz. can	3.2	3.2
Instant Breakfast Drinks		
Start	2.8	1.0
Awake	3.0	1.2
Tang	3.8	1.4
	(5 oz.)	
Tomato Juice, cans, bottles		
A & P, 46-oz. can	3.5	3.6
Campbell, 46-oz. can	4.5	4.7
Welch, 32-oz. bottle	5.5	5.7
Campbell, 12-oz. can	6.3	6.5
	(6 oz.)	
Orange Drinks, 46-oz. can		
Bohack	3.6	3.6
Del Monte	3.9	3.9
A & P	4.2	4.2
Hi-C	4.8	4.8
Hi-C, 12-oz. can	6.0	6.0
Welch	5.1	5.1
Cranberry Juice Drink		
Ocean Spray, 32-oz. bottle	10.8	10.8
Lemonade, made with frozen concentrate		
Private Brand	2.3	6.6
Minute Maid	2.8	8.2
Lemonade, canned, with added vit. C		
Stokely, 46-oz. can	4.3	4.3
Lemonade, made from bottled lemon juice		
Sunkist	2.0	5.8
Realemon	2.3	6.6

	Usual Serving Costs	30 mgs. Vit. C Costs
	(8 oz.)	
Hawaiian Punch		
Orange	6.8¢	6.8¢
Soft Drink Mixes		
Funny Face	1.9	5.6
Kool-Aid	3.3	9.8

*Regional chains, but most supermarkets now have similar "own brand" orange juice. In fact, the same Florida packer puts up frozen concentrate for most chains under their own names.

**Tomato juice has about half the vitamin C of orange juice, but is higher in vitamin A. Pineapple juice listed has vitamin C added to provide 30 mgs. per 4-oz. serving. New formula distributed in 1971 has higher vitamin C content, as noted in text, and cost of 30 mgs. would be comparatively lower; for example, 1.7 cents based on a retail price of 39 cents for a 46-ounce can.

Some "C-Rich" Fruits and Vegetables	Milligrams per Listed Portion
Cantaloupe, one-half (385 grams)	63
Grapefruit, one-half (285 grams)	50
Orange (180-210 grams)	66-75
Strawberries, 1 cup (149 grams)	87
Broccoli spears, cooked, 1 cup (150 grams)	111
Brussels sprouts, cooked, 1 cup (130 grams)	61
Cabbage, 1 cup:	
Shredded, raw (100 grams)	50
Cooked, small amount water, short time (170 grams)	53
Cooked, large amount water, long time (170 grams)	32
Sauerkraut, canned (150 grams)	24

Some "C-Rich" Fruits and Vegetables	Milligrams per Listed Portion
Collards, cooked, 1 cup (190 grams)	84
Kale, cooked, 1 cup (110 grams)	56
Potato, medium:	
Baked or boiled with skin on (136 grams)	22
Peeled, then boiled (122 grams)	20
Spinach, cooked, 1 cup (180 grams)	54
Sweet potato, peeled after cooking (120 grams)	24
Tomato:	
1 medium, raw (150 grams)	35
1 cup, canned or cooked (242 grams)	40
Turnip greens, cooked, 1 cup (145 grams)	87

8

WHAT DO YOU EXPECT, EGG IN YOUR "EGG BREAD"?

The price of bread has become a source of concern both to families and government authorities. The government agencies are sensitive to the impact of this staple on general living costs, to the price-fixing that sometimes has been discovered and to the question often raised about the nutritional quality of bread.

Ordinary white bread, in fact, did go up from 1960 to 1970 at a 22 percent faster rate than the average increase on other foods. Curiously, the price of white bread has jumped noticeably more than that of other cereals and bakery products, and of the ingredients themselves.

Not that the cost of the ingredients really affects the price of bread today. Back in the 1947-49 period the farmer got 3.3 cents for the wheat and other ingredients that go into a 1-pound loaf of bread. The bread sold at retail for 12.7 cents. Now the farmer gets 4 cents for the ingredients and the bread sells for 24.5 cents. The cost of the ingredients went up approximately 21 percent, the price of the bread, 93 percent. If the farmer gave away the wheat and other ingredients in a 25-cent loaf, it would still cost you 21 cents.

When Betty Furness was serving in 1968 as the White House consumer assistant, she observed that bread and bread alone had accounted for nearly a fifth of the total increase in grocery store prices in the previous twenty-five years. She showed the damage that can be done by price-fixing, as in the classic case in the 1950's when the leading wholesale bakers and the largest grocery chain in Washington were found guilty of conspiring to fix both the wholesale and retail prices.

Miss Furness reported that "their closed-door sessions in a Seattle athletic club" managed to drive the price in that area to 19 percent above the national average, and to 20 percent above what it had been in Washington before the price-fixing started. (Interestingly, bread prices in Seattle now are about 11 percent *below* the national average.)

This is not to say that the price of bread always or often is fixed, by a band of well-nourished executives hiding in a club locker room. But there have been other cases of rigging the price of this basic food, as in a conviction in Philadelphia in 1963. A number of bakers there had conspired to fix the price of "economy bread," which is bread usually sold under different brand names by stores for less than the prices of the so-called standard brands. Altogether, the FTC brought nine price conspiracy cases against bakers in the decade from 1959-69, its former chief economist, Willard F. Mueller, has reported.

Significantly, Mueller points out, it is usually not possible for local bakers to fix prices unless the large local retailers go along. Otherwise, their private brands in effect put a ceiling on the prices that the wholesale bakers can charge. In the Washington price conspiracy, only one member of the group was allowed to deviate from the prices set by the association, Mueller reports. This was the dominant grocery chain in Seattle, Safeway Stores, which had its own bakery.

The FTC's record showed that "while the other bakers were urged to retail their bread for the same price that Continental [the largest wholesale baker in Seattle] got for its Wonder bread," Safeway was permitted to sell for 1 cent less. The FTC also found that each time the baker acting as the price leader raised his price, the others followed quickly, often on the same date.

But after the FTC's 1964 decision breaking up the conspiracy, the price of Safeway's bread tumbled, until by 1966 it was selling its brand at 7 cents below the wholesale bakers' brands, or 26 percent below the price that would have existed had the 1-cent differential been maintained, according to Mueller.

The more basic reason for the high cost of bread and the especially rapid increase in the price in the past ten years, is the proliferation of many different types of bread and the cost of marketing them. There now are over twenty different varieties of bread in general production, plus numerous other specialty products such as different types of rolls. The number of sizes has increased too. The House Agricultural Subcommittee found one large chain baked 150 different types and sizes of breads.

In four supermarkets in just one eastern city our own survey found actually thirty-one different types of bread, from white to orange raisin bread. We also found twelve different weights, ranging from 7 to 32 ounces.

The cost of distributing this unnecessary and largely unwanted proliferation of breads is the real motive power behind the accelerated rise in prices. Bread distribution involves an expensive duplicating delivery system, with a half-dozen or more baker-wholesalers delivering to each store each day. With a number of bakers delivering to each store, each delivers fewer loaves and delivery costs rise geometrically. For example, the Quality Bakers of America Cooperative found that a routeman took only twenty-eight minutes to deliver and shelf-load 183 units, but needed seven minutes for twenty-four loaves at a delivery cost per loaf of almost twice as much. The many different types he now handles also slows down the salesman. In fact, the average bread salesman-driver now delivers only about two-thirds the amount on his route that he was able to distribute twenty years ago, W. G. Held, of the U.S. Agriculture Department, has reported. The proliferation also has increased the returns of stale bread.

It costs almost as much to bring bread from the baking plant to your shopping cart as it does to grow the wheat, mill the flour and bake the bread.

The retailers margin of 4 to 5 cents on a 25-cent loaf of bread alone is higher than the farm cost of the ingredients.

Many large retailers now offer their own brands of bread, baked either in their own bakeries or packaged for them by wholesale bakers who also have their own advertised brands. These private brands often sell for 4 to 11 cents less than the equivalent breads under advertised names. Actually the differential on private-brand breads of some retailers is less than it could be. When prices of advertised or regional brands rise, so do those of the private brands, even though the retailers who have private-brand breads do not experience as heavy sales and delivery costs, Federal Trade Commissioner Mary Gardiner Jones has pointed out.

Some retailers really cut the price of private-brand breads, selling them for as much as 11 cents a pound less than the advertised brands. Other retailers peg their price only 3 or 4 cents below the advertised brands. In Canada in 1968, labor and farm groups protesting an increase in the price of bread to as much as 29 cents, pointed out that a co-op bakery was able to sell bread for 17 cents, the *Maritime Cooperator* reported.

Adding to the consumer's confusion in trying to buy best value in bread is the trend to multiple pricing, such as three loaves for 89 cents, and the juggling around of weights. For example, after the New York Legislature in 1967 repealed its law requiring that bread be packaged in even sizes, a variety of new sizes appeared, with bread now sold in such weights as 7, 8, 11, 14, 16, 20, 22, 24 and 32 ounces. The proliferation of sizes also has made it possible for bakers to reduce weights; for example, from 22 to 20 ounces.

For the consumer the result is a great deal of expensive confusion, and some noticeable foolery both in the special varieties and the size appearance of bread.

You can pay as much as 45 cents a pound for "egg bread," 35 cents a pound for "cheese bread" or a nickel more a loaf for "potato bread," and you know what? You'll probably be getting much the same bread as if you paid 24 to 26 cents a pound for ordinary white bread.

The fact is, there are no standards for all the special breads. Only ordinary white bread, whole wheat bread, enriched bread, milk bread and raisin bread must meet minimum government specifications for ingredients. A baker can put as much or as little egg as he wants into an "egg bread," as much or as little butter into "butter bread," as much or as little "buttermilk" into "buttermilk bread," and so on.

For some unknown reason, unless because it is a different shape, you also may pay 10 or 15 percent more for some brands of "sandwich bread" than for the same baker's ordinary white bread. Or if you buy white bread in a round shape instead of rectangular, you can pay 35 cents a pound instead of 25. You may even find yourself paying 10 percent more per pound for "thin-sliced" bread than for the same bread in the standard loaf.

Moreover, the "truth-in-packaging" law is not too much help when it comes to bread. Except in a few states that require standard loaves, such as a pound, you still have to try to compare the cost per pound of a 16-ounce loaf of white bread at two for 45 cents, with a 20-ounce loaf for 30 cents, a 22-ounce loaf for 37, a 29-ounce for 51, and a 32-ounce loaf for 59. In this particular case, the smaller 16-, 20- and 22-ounce loaves cost less per pound than the larger sizes, although this is not necessarily always true.

But compare you must. You can pay anywhere from 23 to 32 cents a pound for white bread, and up to 39 or more for "diet" and other special types.

There no longer seems to be any particular logic in the way the stores price even ordinary bread. One supermarket may charge more for sandwich bread than for ordinary white. Another may charge the same. One store may charge less per pound for larger loaves; another may charge the same or more. A "special" can throw your previous figuring off completely.

There really is only one solution to this money-wasting confusion. If the government can't get bakers to standardize the size of loaves, then in all fairness stores should be required to state the cost per pound as well as the price of the loaf, just as they usually do with meat.

The Food and Drug Administration itself is concerned about the lack of standards for specialty breads. There is no doubt that the public is either being misled or is fooling itself. James O. Dunston, FDA food technologist, reports, for example, that consumers questioned in a survey often believed that a loaf of egg bread has two eggs. Another large group estimated one egg, and a third group, three or more eggs.

But the seventeen so-called "egg breads" analyzed by FDA actually contained only one-fifth of an egg to about 1½ eggs, with a frequency high of one-third of an egg, and an average of slightly more than half an egg, Dunston noted.

In contrast, we found some brands of egg bread selling for

almost twice as much as ordinary bread, or as much as 20-22 cents extra. For 22 cents you can buy four eggs.

The public also is far from reality in what it thinks it gets in butter bread. The FDA found that at least one brand of "butter bread" had no butter at all. The average was slightly more than 1½ pats of butter. In contrast, 20 percent of the users surveyed expected eight pats (slices). The actual 1½ pats is three-eighths of an ounce, or about 2 cents worth of butter.

With "potato bread," too, the survey found that the public expects to get as much as 10 ounces of potato flour in such bread. They actually get an average of about a half ounce.

In fact, Dunston points out, ordinary white bread is permitted to have up to 3 percent of potato flour, about a third of an ounce, as an optional ingredient. So, some of the so-called potato breads are not much different from plain white bread.

Buttermilk bread is the only special brand checked which almost approximated the amount of buttermilk the public believes it has. The consumers tended to estimate 8 fluid ounces of buttermilk. The actual average found by the FDA was 5 ounces. But you can't depend on it. Some brands had less than a half ounce. Others had as much as 9. But there is no way for the consumer to tell in the present absence of standards or informative labeling.

As long ago as 1948 FDA sought to establish standards for these various special breads. The bakers insisted on much lower standards than the government agency wanted. For example, FDA proposed at least 5 percent egg solids by weight of flour in egg bread. That is less than half an egg, and low enough. The bakers proposed no more than 2 percent, or one-sixth of an egg. For all the nutritional value, you may as well have no egg at all. The yellow hue of "egg bread" usually comes from added coloring, not from added eggs.

Similarly, FDA wanted at least 12 percent milk fat from butter in "butter bread," with this as the only shortening. A baker's trade organization wanted the minimum to be only 4 percent.

The net effect is that not only has the price of even standard bread gone up out of proportion to those of other foods from grains and cereals and to food costs as a whole,[11] but consumers are further raising their own costs by buying the more expensive specialty types and buns and rolls. For example, hamburger buns and other types of rolls have become a big seller. While bread in the form of ordinary white loaves may be 25 cents a pound (the national average) in the form of hamburger buns, hero loaves, frankfurter and other types of rolls, the cost becomes 50-60 cents.

The Illusion of Size

The appearance of size can be another cost-raiser. In the survey for this book we found, for example, three brands that appeared to be the same size but were labeled 22, 29 and 32 ounces. The difference in volume for the same weight occurs because some bread has more air per pound. Baking companies achieve this by, for example, baking 1 pound of ingredients in a 1 ½-pound pan.

Yet, despite the fact that in some markets balloon bread costs as much as 5 cents more per pound than the standard loaf, it is now the leading seller in stores that stock it, the USDA's *Farm Index* reports.

This is a shocker because all that housewives need do is look at the weight marked on the wrapper and compare the price per pound with other breads, even though some arithmetic is involved because of the varying weights.

Balloon bread is most widely sold on the West Coast. At least two states—Oregon and Arizona—now require that it be labeled as such, despite losing court battles by bakers to prevent state authorities from requiring such labeling. While the modern fluffy or puffy white breads sold in the East are not ballooned to as great an extent, the difference in the volume between various brands has become increasingly noticeable, with the increase in the size of the pans used by commercial bakers. You can observe the difference yourself by squeezing some of the largest-looking loaves.

You may feel that balloon or other fluffy or puffy bread is suitable for your purposes. The USDA did find in one test that some of the test group preferred fluffy bread that had a volume of ten cubic inches per ounce, compared with bread that had seven cubic inches. But you still need to make sure that you do not pay more for the illusion of size.

Nor can you trust a name. Such designations on various brands as Jumbo, Giant, Extra Large, King Size, Big Loafer, Mr. Big and Big Boy have no meaning at all in an era of varying weights and expanded volume.

The Nutritional Question

The nutritional quality of bread also has become a matter of concern and contention. Thirty-one states require that white bread be enriched by the addition of the B vitamins (thiamine, riboflavin, niacin) and iron, with calcium and vitamin D as optional additions. Such enrichment restores the B vitamins and iron lost in milling the original whole wheat. In the states that do not require it, many breads are enriched voluntarily by bakers. The breads that may not be enriched actually may be the more expensive specialty breads, and, rather disturbingly, the hamburger buns and doughnuts favored by youngsters.

The states that do not require enrichment are chiefly those in the West. Home economists at the Berkeley co-ops in California campaigned for five years for mandatory enrichment in that state, and finally in 1970 the state legislature enacted the necessary law. The additional cost to the baker was estimated to be less than a half cent a loaf.

Cake flours also can use enrichment, since these are the most finely ground and are low in protein. (Pasta flours are milled from durum wheat and are relatively high in protein.)

Because of these gaps, mandatory enrichment by federal law of all flour at the mill has been proposed. This would be a useful step in assuring the nutritional value of bread and other wheat products. But until this is done you can make sure by looking for the "enriched" description, and, if available in your area, the listing of the amount of the B vitamins, iron and other added nutrients supplied by different types and brands of bread. These vary. Some may supply more than the minimum.

But some nutritionists feel that the nourishment in bread should be increased beyond "enrichment." The Food and Drug Administration has recommended that the level of iron in enriched bread be increased to meet the recommendations of nutritionists who have concluded that much of our population is receiving too little iron in its regular diet, reports Douglass L. Mann, president of the American Bakers Association.

While "enrichment" puts back at least the nutrients considered most essential and so restores a food to the natural level of the original product, "fortification" means adding ingredients to provide certain nutrients which may not be naturally present, Theresa Demus, director of FDA Consumer Services, explains. Thus, in recent years, the proportion of milk solids in a typical loaf of white bread has been increased to 4 percent. This has been an inexpensive way to provide additional protein and calcium, and especially useful in that the protein is the more complete kind, from an animal source.

There have been proposals to raise the proportion of milk solids further—to 6 or even 8 percent. One fortified bread, known as the Cornell formula or McKay bread (after its developer, Clive W. McKay), used a combination of 8 percent nonfat milk solids, 6 percent soybean flour and 2 percent wheat germ for a high-protein loaf. However, the Cornell formula bread currently is reported to be used only by a few small bakers because of its extra cost.

Tests by the U.S. Agriculture Department did find that users preferred bread made with at least 4 percent milk solids to bread with no milk solids, and bread with 8 percent milk had even some further preference over the 4 percent. (The consumers in the test indicated their preference without knowing what ingredients were used in the sample breads.) Fortification of bread is a more economical and surer way to provide additional nutrients than fortification of high-priced breakfast cereals.

At the very least, the baking industry and the Food and Drug Administration owe the consuming public what is known as "open formula" labeling. This would include the facts on all the ingredients used in the bread, the quantities of these ingredients and the percentage of protein. Then at least we can know what each brand or type offers and select whatever best suits our needs or preferences. This would be the real "free choice" that the food industry always claims the consumer has, though he actually does not, when he lacks the information to choose.

Consumers are not, of course, seeking old-fashioned drastic remedies. A couple of hundred years ago, a baker in Turkey or Egypt who sold light or adulterated bread (the balloon bread of the eighteenth century) was punished by having his ear nailed to his shop door. All we are asking is that balloon bread be labeled as such, and that all the facts about ingredients be shown clearly on the wrapper.

The Money-Saving Way

Pending improvements in labeling and merchandising, all you can do now is use these facts:

1. Standard bread costs the least.

2. The larger sizes often save as much as 8 percent of the cost. (But look at the weights; don't depend on appearances.)

3. The private brands cost less.

9

THE MAGIC ABACUS OF
THE MEAT PACKERS

Meat is the single most expensive item in your food budget. Yet meat has become one of the most confusing items to buy, with prices, weights, quality and even names of cuts frequently juggled, and value often cheapened with added fat and water.

Fat Franks and Wet Bologna

Franks and luncheon meats have become one of the most notorious areas of quality and price manipulation. Faced in a typical supermarket by, as we found in one, 127 types, brands and package sizes of lunch meats plus 25 types and sizes of canned lunch meats and 12 kinds and sizes of franks, you can find yourself paying a couple of dollars a pound for lunch meat without realizing it or buying lunch "meats" and franks that are really only half meat.

Franks and lunch meats are permitted to have up to 30 percent added fat and 10 percent added water. There was a furor in 1969 when the Agriculture Department proposed to officially permit meat packers to put as much as 33 percent fat in frankfurters.

The department had found that nationally the average fat content had risen that high. So the department felt it might as well legitimize this average and make it the maximum. The range of fat content it found was 14 percent to 51 percent.

But the USDA ran into opposition. Virginia Knauer, the consumer assistant to the president, said 33 percent was too much. She wanted to hold the line at 30 percent. The Consumer Federation of America and the National Consumers League wanted to roll back the limit to 25 percent.

The fat content had been sneaking up since the average 14 percent in 1945. As more fat was added, the food value in terms of protein had declined from 15 percent in 1945 to 11.7 percent in 1968, with most of the decrease actually occurring after 1955.

USDA officials argued that a lower limit would necessitate the use of more lean meat at a cost of about 2 cents more per pound, including control costs, and consumers would have to pay an additional price. This is either an unthinking or specious argument. Consumers then could get the same protein and vitamin value from correspondingly less sausage, and if they wanted more fat, could merely consume a little margarine at 25 cents a pound rather than pay 80 cents or more for it in franks.

The industry claims the public wants these "juicier" franks. I have received thousands of letters and verbal complaints from consumers during thirty years in this work, but have never heard a consumer demand juicier franks. (Purported consumers "demand" for "juicier" franks also has been made the excuse for adding up to 10 percent water to modern cured hams.)

The domination by industry of the Agriculture Department standards policies came to light at the 1969 House hearings on food labeling when Congressman Rosenthal disclosed a USDA document which said: "As you are aware, in 1958 the Department attempted to limit fat content to 30 percent. This met stiff opposition from industry and was withdrawn from enforcement."

High fat limits penalize the scrupulous producer who keeps fat content low and legitimizes the producer who uses a lot of fat in franks and bologna, Rosenthal observed. In further fact, high limits tend to push a producer who would rather make leaner franks into using more fat because of competitive pressures.

That consumers have not been aware of the climbing percentage of fat in such processed meats is shown by a survey the Agriculture Department itself made. It found the public thinks there is less fat than there really is, Mrs. Knauer pointed out.

The food manufacturers are able to get away with adding extra fat by a new method of emulsifying it so it doesn't separate in cooking and you can't see it. What you think is a nice juicy frank is really a nice fatty and watery one.

The water is added in the form of cold water and chopped ice when the meat is being ground for frankfurters, bologna, cooked salami and similar luncheon meats. The claim is that the water and ice are needed to keep the ground meat cool in this stage of preparation and "add moisture for good texture and consistency." But it remains in the meat and you pay for it. If you try to fry a slice of modern bologna you can see for yourself the water in the pan just as you can see the fat boil out of a modern frank.

The battle over how much fat the government should permit in franks reveals how the present system of standards for food products fools the public. If manufacturers and the Agriculture Department were 100 percent honest with the public, they would say on the label the percentages of meat, fat and water. If we oppose 33 percent fat but say it's all right to hide 30 percent or even 25 percent in these products without telling the public, we are saying it is all right to fool the public a lot, but don't fool us this 10 percent more.

The actual average fat content of franks, bologna and other sausages in mid-1970 was 27 percent, the department has reported.

But the USDA has been loath to reveal its data on fat content of different brands. The *Detroit Free Press* had to appeal to interested congressmen and the Agriculture Secretary to pry loose some of this information. Reporter Trudy Lieberman revealed that franks from such big packers as Armour, Swift, Wilson, and Hormel ranged around the 30 percent limit in early 1970. One packer, Hygrade, had reduced its fat content to 20 percent. Many of the specialty and kosher franks averaged about 24 percent, Miss Lieberman noted.

The worst kidding is "All Beef" or "All Meat" frankfurters and bologna. They are not "all meat" at all. They are usually close to 30 percent fat and 10 percent water, plus 2 percent corn syrup, flavoring ingredients and preservatives. Thus, they are really about 50 percent meat.

If you look at the label on "All Beef Frankfurters" you will see it states "Beef, water, salt," and so on. "All Meat" franks, bologna and similar luncheon meats may say "Beef, pork, water, salt," etc. Just plain "Franks" or other processed meats may say "Beef, pork, water, nonfat dry milk, cereal," etc.

Actually the less-expensive plain franks and luncheon meats not labeled "All Beef" or "All Meat" are the better buy, both nutritionally and economically. Not only do they cost less, but the addition of nonfat milk and cereals increase their protein value.

"All Meat" franks have 59.4 grams of protein per pound. So do franks with added nonfat milk. Franks with cereal added have 65.3 grams. Franks with both cereal and nonfat milk added have 64.4 grams. The regulations permit 3 ½ percent of cereal or nonfat milk to be added to franks and luncheon meats, and this is certainly preferable to more fat.

So here's a case where the cheapest is actually the best.

Note also the standards for liver sausage products in the standards list in the Appendix. Only 30 percent liver content is required.

Franks and lunch meats are not the only meats with added water nowadays. Many hams are cured in a pickle solution of curing ingredients and water injected into them. Those labeled "water added" have up to 10 percent added water after curing. If more, the ham must be labeled "imitation ham."

The Weight Jugglers

The manipulation of weights of prepackaged luncheon meats can be as costly to you as the manipulation of the quality inside the package. You need a magic abacus of your own to compare relative values among seven different-sized packages of bologna, six different weights of liver sausage, and eight different weights of salami.

In all, in one supermarket we found sixteen different sizes of prepackaged lunch meats, ranging from 3 to 18 ½ ounces. These included such potentially misleading oddities as 3 ½ ounces, 3 ¾,

4½, 5, 13 and the ubiquitous 14-ounce packages instead of an old-fashioned 16-ounce pound.

It is difficult enough to estimate in your head the comparative value of the same brand's 5-ounce package of bologna for 45 cents against its 7-ounce package for 59 cents. But under the present circumstances you also have to compare a 3¼-ounce package of sliced ham at 59 cents with one of 4¼-ounces at 69 cents. (The answer is given in the table of typical lunch meat prices in this chapter.)

The juggling of weights may not seem as illogical to the packer as to you. One packer sells 8-ounce bulk pieces of braunschweiger for 43 cents. His sliced package is 9 ounces for 61 cents. Unless you stop to figure the cost per pound, you will not realize that you pay for the bulk package at the rate of 86 cents a pound, but for the sliced at the rate of $1.08.

Note especially the much higher costs of the same lunch meats sliced as shown in the charts, and the especially high costs of small packages. A 4½-ounce package of bologna for 39 cents comes to $1.39 a pound; an 8-ounce package at 52 cents comes to $1.04; a 14-ounce bulk piece is only 69 cents. Unsliced lunch meats also keep better in your refrigerator.

But the magic abacus is at its most profitable when packers combine lunch meats and cheese or several types of lunch meats in a variety or combination pack. If you buy 8 ounces of pimento cheese for 53 cents and 8 ounces of lunch meat for 57 cents, the pound cost would be $1.10. If a packer puts them together in one package, you may find the per-pound rate is $1.39.

Because of concern over both freshness and price, more shoppers have begun to buy lunch meats at supermarket deli counters. Our comparison indicates that the prices are no higher for these freshly sliced lunch meats and cheese, and in fact are less costly than brand-name prepackaged varieties.

The Case of the Ruddy Hamburger

One frankly deceptive—not merely manipulative—trick is the addition of excessive amounts of fat to hamburger. Some stores color high-fat hamburger by adding beef blood. The butcher's real prize is the large blood clot often found in beef fat. This goes right into the grinder.

Markets often run chopped beef through the grinder several times to make it look as red as possible. The extra grindings more thoroughly blend the fat with the lean. The butcher may be under economic pressure from several directions—first, to show a profit, especially in times of high meat prices when stores must still offer specials; also, to make the meat department take in enough extra to cover meat taken home by employees, including himself, or pilferage by customers.

Butchers also have used—or still use—paprika, a weak-flavored pepper—to preserve the color in meat that has begun to spoil, as well as to make it appear leaner than it really is. In 1969, the USDA banned the practice, at least officially.

Federal standards require that hamburger must contain no more than 30 percent fat. But state regulations can vary considerably. The use of beef blood and paprika to color hamburger is not harmful to health, but is certainly a financial deception.

Some meat sellers and restaurants also add cereal and soybean derivatives, which at least provide better-quality nutrients than added fat, but are neither as complete in protein nor as valuable as meat itself.

Another dangerous practice is the addition of pork scraps to hamburger. Some families like to cook their hamburger rare. But pork needs longer cooking.

As well as hamburger, carefully inspect the veal and other patties sold by markets nowadays, under the name of "veal birds," "mock chicken leg," etc. Such patties have in many instances become a way of unloading meat scraps ground up with extra suet.

The most dubious purchase is already prepared hamburger portions, sold plain or in stuffed cabbage, stuffed peppers, and similar products. One market manager explained that this all-purpose chopped meat was prepared by first soaking it in water, and then adding seasonings. Thus customers pay higher prices for a product that is part water and seasonings.

In Kansas, a consumer leader, Diane Goertz, warned consumers and beef producers of proposals to permit the sale of "beef patties," to which packers could add any desired amount of binders or extenders such as wheat, oatmeal or soybeans. At this writing, the proposal is still pending. She also warned against a proposed change in state regulations, which would permit breading ⁄on "beef patties" or "fabricated steaks." The content of such a product, she pointed out, would be 30 percent breading, 21 percent fat, and 49 percent beef.

Higher Costs, Shorter Weights

Judging from reports from several regions, when meat prices are high, either the incidence of shortweighting increases or consumers check more carefully. In New York City, complaints about short weights on packaged meats almost doubled in 1969, reported Consumer Commissioner Bess Myerson Grant.

Markets department reports from Ohio, Vermont, Virginia and other areas indicate short weights may be more prevalent than we realize. They can occur in any type of supermarket—national chains as well as smaller stores. In Nassau County, New York, Consumer Commissioner John Occhiogrosso reported meat short weights were the second largest class of short weight, exceeded only by short weights in macaroni products.

Dr. Leland Gordon, director of the Weights and Measures Research Center at Denison University, reports that in state after state he was told that the largest number of shortages was found in meat stores and departments, sometimes because of carelessness due to heavy workloads, sometimes because of management pressure to show good returns.

A Vermont inspector, John Granger, warned consumers they may be losing as much as 25 or 30 cents through short weights every time they go shopping, although he also said many of the errors may be due to carelessness. [12]

Mislabeling and Nonlabeling

Another growing practice, especially in times of high prices, is that of cutting standard cuts of meat such as chuck and roasts into steaks of different shapes and calling them by other names. Thus, such steaks as "fillet steak," "breakfast steak," "king steak," "London broil," and other glamorized names.

Similarly, "cross cut rib roast" in some parts of the country may be cut from the blade section of the chuck, and elsewhere, from the shoulder arm portion of the chuck. In either case, it is chuck, not rib roast, as the name might imply.

Our experience is that such different cuts usually cost about 20 cents a pound more than the original chuck. Stores also often charge 5 to 10 cents more a pound for boneless stew cut from the chuck than for the parent boneless chuck roast.

Apparently the younger consumers are attracted to the romantically named steaks. In one store a young woman advised another not to buy a regular-sized sirloin steak but the "cute-looking his 'n her steaks." An Indiana meat manager confided to a *Supermarket News* reporter that new names for old steaks have become widely used because young homemakers today do not understand what a "crown roast" is. But they know how they live and understand such terms as "patio steaks" and "pizza burgers." They are looking for convenience and prepared foods more than their parents did, he explained.

But romance is not without its cost. Wanda Mead, Nassau County extension home economist, pointed out that a "club steak" may come from the rib or the chuck, and the price should be proportionate.[13]

In some states stores must name in ads and on labels the primal cut as well as the fanciful name. Other areas make no such requirement—the buyer must fend for himself.

This is what Occhiogrosso calls "nonlabeling." But there also are instances of actual mislabeling. Four Nassau County chain supermarkets were enjoined in 1970 from such practices as selling round steak worth $1.18 a pound as "sirloin steak fillet" at $1.79 and chuck steak worth $1.09 to $1.29 as "minute steak round" at $1.59 a pound. Complaints against six other stores were settled by administrative agreement to stop any such practices. Of forty stores that were checked by the Nassau County consumer department, actually thirty-eight had some instance of mislabeling or nonlabeling.

But buying costly grades may be the biggest fooler of all. The expensive "Choice" grade does not have as much lean as the cheaper "Good" and "Standard" grades, as explained in Chapter 17. Thus, it does not have as much protein, and so is less nutritious. For example, assuming the same trim, a "Choice" round roast has 76 percent separable lean, the "Good" grade, 80, and the "Standard," 86. Nowadays these lower grades can be broiled and the consumer no longer has to rely on moist cooking to make them tender.

THE REAL COSTS OF LUNCH MEATS*

(Sliced, except as noted)

	Unit Net Wt.	Price of Unit	Cost per Lb.
Luncheon Meat and Loaf			
Co-op can	12 oz.	$.61	$ .81
Hormel Spam, can	12	.65	.87
Made Rite	8	.59	1.18
Bob Ostrow	7	.59	1.35
Oscar Mayer	8	.68	1.36
Bob Ostrow	5	.43	1.38
Capri	4	.39	1.56
Summer Sausage			
Dubuque Royal Buffet, unsliced, bulk pieces	—	—	1.29
Dubuque Royal Buffet, unsliced	12	.98	1.31
Oscar Mayer	8	.79	1.58
Olive Loaf			
Oscar Mayer	8	.67	1.34
Bob Ostrow	5	.43	1.38
Thuringer			
Saag's, unsliced, bulk pieces	—	—	1.59
Hormel, unsliced	7	.75	1.71
Hormel	4	.49	1.96
Pepperoni			
Rath, unsliced	7½	.75	1.60
Hormel	3½	.59	2.70

	Unit Net Wt.	Price of Unit	Cost per Lb.
Salami			
Cooked			
Co-op, unsliced, bulk pieces	— oz.	$ —	$ .79
Rath	16	.89	.89
Made Rite	8	.59	1.18
Morrell	8	.59	1.18
Oscar Mayer	8	.64	1.28
Bob Ostrow	7	.59	1.35
Bob Ostrow	5	.45	1.44
Gallo	5	.49	1.57
Beef			
Allan's, unsliced	16	.99	.99
Oscar Mayer	8	.67	1.34
Best's kosher, unsliced	12	1.12	1.49
H & S, unsliced	16	1.49	1.49
Gallo	5	.67	2.14
Dry			
Gallo, unsliced	13	1.39	1.71
Gallo, unsliced	8	.97	1.94
Capri, unsliced	12	1.49	1.99
Capri, unsliced	8	1.09	2.18
Gallo	6	.86	2.29
Capri	6	.98	2.61
Gallo	3	.55	2.93
Capri	3	.55	2.93
Bologna			
Beef & Pork			
Co-op, unsliced, bulk pieces	—	—	.69
Allan's, unsliced	16	.75	.75
Made Rite	14	.79	.91
Oscar Mayer	12	.69	.92
Oscar Mayer	8	.52	1.04
Bob Ostrow	12	.79	1.05
Capri	10	.69	1.10
Capri	4½	.39	1.39
Beef			
Made Rite	14	.79	.90
Oscar Mayer	12	.73	.97

	Unit Net Wt.	Price of Unit	Cost per Lb.
Oscar Mayer	8 oz.	$ .54	$1.08
Morrell	8	.55	1.10
Made Rite	8	.59	1.18
H & S, unsliced	16	1.19	1.19
Bob Ostrow	7	.59	1.35
Bob Ostrow	5	.45	1.44

Ham

Danola	4¼	.69	2.60
Capri	4	.69	2.76
Leo's	4	.69	2.76
Bob Ostrow	3¼	.59	2.90
Chopped			
Hormel, can	12	.83	1.11
Oscar Mayer	8	.86	1.72
Danola	4	.49	1.96
Bob Ostrow	4	.49	1.96
Leo's, pressed	3	.39	2.08
Carl Buddig, pressed	3	.39	2.08
Leo's	3½	.49	2.24
Capri	4	.59	2.36

Liver Sausage

Allan's braunschweiger, unsliced, bulk pieces	—	—	.75
Oscar Mayer braunschweiger, unsliced	8	.43	.86
Oscar Mayer braunschweiger, unsliced	4	.24	.96
Oscar Mayer braunschweiger	9	.61	1.08
Saag's smoked braunschweiger, unsliced, bulk pieces	—	—	1.25
Bob Ostrow liver loaf	6	.49	1.31
Oscar Mayer liver cheese	8	.67	1.34

---

*Adapted from unit pricing charts of Berkeley, California, Consumers Cooperative, December, 1969.

CHAPTER

10

POULTRY: DIVIDED, WATERED AND STUFFED

Like many other foods today, broilers, turkey and other poultry often are watered, cut into parts, sold with additional ingredients and with added fat—all at disproportionately higher prices.

Most poultry sold today is frozen, and you do get extra water with frozen poultry—as much as 8 percent legally but sometimes more. The water is absorbed in the chicken when it is given an ice-water bath to chill it before freezing.

Paying poultry prices for even the permissible 8 percent of added water is serious enough. Based on an estimate by the government's General Accounting Office, consumers pay in the neighborhood of $250 million a year for the legally added water, or at the rate of $33 million for each increase of 1 percent in weight, Sue Hoover reported in the Detroit *News*. If you buy, say, two frozen broilers a week, you may be paying about $25 a year for the water, perhaps even more.

But much poultry comes on the market with even more than the permitted 8 percent. In some packing plants the government investigators found that over 20 percent of the chickens shipped had more than 8 percent because of inadequate government supervision. The plants simply do not drain the poultry sufficiently before freezing and packing.

The injection of water is one reason why people often feel

chicken does not taste as good as it used to, even though they may not realize why.

The sogginess of modern frozen broilers even has proved to be a problem for exporters in selling them to European countries. The Europeans like to drink their water separately.

What can you do about the watered chickens? The only truly effective remedy can come from the Agriculture Department through reduction of the present 8 percent allowance to a fairer, less money-wasting limit *and* firm regulation of that limit.

But if you are alerted by this report, you can watch for poultry that appears especially soggy when you defrost it, and you can notify the store and also avoid that brand. Younger, lighter, more tender birds such as broilers tend to absorb more water than older, heavier ones such as fowl.

You also can be misled into paying excessive prices by the now widespread merchandising practice of selling poultry in parts. The price is disproportionately higher for two reasons. One is that stores find it more difficult to dispose of the less wanted parts, such as the backs and wings. Also, in general, stores take a higher profit margin on the parts.

Note the chart in this chapter, listing the prices at which parts would be an equally good buy at various price levels for a whole broiler-fryer. We checked prices in three cities to see if stores do price parts in line with their value.

In not one store or city did we find that stores price parts anywhere near the relative value of the price of the whole chicken. Some charged a lot extra and some a little. There was no noticeable rational reason for the pricing—apparently, just the store's estimate of what the traffic would bear.

The stores overcharge for drumsticks, especially. In instances where 41-46 cents a pound would be the real relative value, we found some stores charging as much as 89 cents. The overcharges for breasts and thighs are not as severe. In general, thighs, if sold separately, and wings are the most reasonable relative value because they are least in demand.

As the chart shows, breast halves give you the most edible meat, followed by thighs. Thus, even at a few cents more they are worth more than drumsticks, which have less meat. In one fairly typical example, we found whole broilers at 43 cents a pound, with the cost of the edible cooked meat thus 83 cents a pound; cut-up breasts were 67 cents, making the edible meat $1.06 a pound, and cut-up legs were 62 cents with the edible meat, $1.16. Wings yield least meat, but stores price them low enough so that they are actually often best value.

But, just as in cars, you cannot assemble a chicken from parts for as little as you can buy the whole chicken.

In general, you can estimate that whole broilers yield 52 percent cooked edible meat; breasts, 63; legs and thighs, 53; wings, 50; backs, 42.

Because backs are harder to get rid of, some stores now sell legs and breasts with a portion of the back left on. These are called "quarters." They should cost at least 10 cents a pound less than the corresponding part.

REAL WORTH OF BROILER PARTS

Parts Are an Equally Good Value if Price Is:

Price of Whole Broiler	Breast Half	Drumstick and Thigh	Drumstick	Thigh	Wing
27¢ lb.	38¢ lb.	35¢ lb.	33¢ lb.	36¢ lb.	21¢ lb.
29	41	37	36	39	23
31	44	40	38	41	25
33	47	42	41	44	26
35	49	45	43	47	28
37	52	47	46	49	29
39	55	50	48	52	31
41	58	53	50	55	33
43	61	55	53	57	34

Price of Whole Broiler	Breast Half	Drumstick and Thigh	Drumstick	Thigh	Wing
45 ¢ lb.	63 ¢ lb.	58 ¢ lb.	55 ¢ lb.	60 ¢ lb.	36 ¢ lb.
47	66	60	58	63	37
49	69	63	60	65	39
51	72	65	63	68	41
53	75	68	65	71	42
55	78	71	68	73	44

Adapted from *Family Economics Review*, U. S. Agriculture Dept.

Packers have found ways to add cheap additional ingredients to turkeys and charge more. The self-basting turkeys really have 3 percent injected fat. It is not butter, as the "butterball" name of one brand may suggest, but coconut oil and water for which you pay a turkey price.

To compound the overcharge, you also pay 5 to 10 cents a pound more for a self-basting turkey. In all, the extra cost for a 12-pound bird will be about $1.20. This saves you about three minutes of actual time expended. So you pay for this time-saving at the rate of $24.80 an hour. If your husband earns less than that, hire him to baste the turkey at a little lower hourly rate. Or if you use aluminum foil or one of the special plastic bags recently developed for roasting, you won't need to do any basting.

The other tricked-up version of turkey at a higher price is the prestuffed kind. As the result of a valiant battle several years ago by Esther Hendler, a New York City markets department inspector, federal regulations now require that in all states the labels must show the amount of stuffing. It usually is about 23 percent of the weight of the bird. Of that amount, about half is the water used to prepare the stuffing.

If you buy a 16-pound prestuffed turkey at 65 cents a pound, figure you are paying about $2.40 for the stuffing. A ready-made packaged stuffing would cost you only about 70 cents, including the fat you add; a home-prepared bread stuffing costs about 55 cents, home economists estimate.

Note also that you get more for your money in big turkeys. They not only cost less per pound (usually about 10 cents less) but yield more meat per pound. A turkey under 16 pounds yields about 50 percent roasted meat; one over 16 pounds yields closer to 55 percent. For a smaller bird, figure you'll need close to three-quarters of a pound of ready-to-cook turkey per person; for a big one, about a half pound.

11

SMALL TRUTHS IN PACKAGING AND THE BATTLE OVER UNIT PRICING

You probably already have noticed in the stores a few changes resulting from the long-sought, hard-fought Truth-in-Packaging, law, which became effective in 1968. All food packages and cans now show the net contents on the front face in fairly large and noticeable type.

Until Congress mandated such clearer labeling you often had to look all over the package for the net weight and even then sometimes could barely read it. There were such examples of hard-to-read weight and ingredient statements as fine glistening print on a curved glistening surface, small black type on a dark green background, silver-colored ink on a white background, and small type perpendicular to the principal display panel.

In a few product lines the previous jungle of many different sizes has been thinned down a little. Also, where manufacturers say how many servings the package provides, they now also say how big the servings are.

For example, in dehydrated mashed potatoes, the packages now specify "8 half-cup servings," or for rice, "12 two-thirds cup servings." This is a help in two ways. The manufacturers now admit how small their concept of a serving may be, such as a half cup of mashed potatoes. Some, in fact, no longer even specify the number of servings on package labels.

When they do, the relative number of same-sized servings

provided by different brands can give you another way to compare values. Obviously, a 21-serving box of French's dehydrated mashed potatoes for 65 cents costs less than an 8-serving box of Hungry Jack mashed for 33 cents (without attempting to compare taste), since both are half-cup servings.

That, however, is most of the benefit so far from the Truth-in-Packaging law. In shopping for most food and toiletry products, you still have to go through a process of dividing the cost per ounce into a large number of package sizes, brands and related varieties.

For example, just one supermarket offers four different brands of tuna fish, each of which comes in three or four types and four or five sizes. This adds up to forty-five different choices. You have to figure out the best buy among 3½ ounces of tuna for 27 cents, 6½ ounces for 37 cents, 7 ounces for 45 cents and 9¼ ounces for 57 cents. In canned sardines you have to compare among such sizes as 1½ ounces, 3¼, 3¾, 4 and 4⅜. Have fun.

We actually found nine different sizes of dehydrated mashed potatoes in just one store, including 5, 5¼, 5½, 6, 8, 13¾, 16 and 16½ ounces.

It still is virtually impossible to compare relative values in baby foods. Just among the meat products for infants and toddlers, we found three different major brands, offering approximately ninety different varieties in four or five different sizes such as 4¼ ounces, 6½ ounces, 7 ounces and so on. Young parents shopping for baby food encounter a terrifying amount of free choice, with a potential of over three hundred different mathematical computations. No wonder the birth rate is beginning to decline.

Among frozen vegetables, we found six different sizes of packages, ranging from 8 to 24 ounces, and with the face of some of the 8- and 9-ounce packages as large as the 10 ounces. An unwary or hurried consumer can be fooled if she doesn't stop to look at the weights.

Even in fresh produce, you can be fooled by the practice of selling some produce by the piece instead of the pound. We weighed six heads of iceberg lettuce, all marked 39 cents, and found they ranged from 13 to 17 ounces. Two buyers get 23 percent less for the same price, depending entirely on chance selection. The same lottery exists in citrus fruits and other produce sold by count rather than weight. For example, in surveying produce departments for this book, Josenhans found honeydew melons all priced 79 cents, but ranging from 4 pounds, 2 ounces to 3 pounds, 14 ounces—a difference of 7 ounces or over 10 percent. He found celery all 35 cents, but ranging from 27 to 21 ounces—a difference of 22 percent. No two of those checked weighed the same.

There is little rhyme or reason in the way fresh fruits are sold. In many areas apples, apricots, bananas, grapes, peaches, pears, cranberries and others are sold by the pound. But oranges, lemons and grapefruit are sold by the count and blueberries and strawberries by volume. Watermelons are sold by weight, honeydews by count.

In vegetables, too, potatoes and carrots are sold by the pound, but sometimes by the carton, and cherry tomatoes by volume. Cabbage is sold by the pound, but cauliflower by the head, and so on. If this is the situation in your locality, and it will be, with only some variations, you will be well-advised to ask your local markets department to seek some sanity by requiring all produce to be sold by the pound, and meanwhile (which could be many years) weigh what you buy on the produce department scales.

Also in shopping for soaps and detergents, you still have a multiplicity of weights. Just among the newly popular deodorant soaps we found soaps in 3½, 3¾, 4¾ and 5-ounce sizes. If you look closely you do get some information. You see, for example, that Dove, which looks like the biggest bar, actually is only 4¾ ounces, and Phase III, 5 ounces, even though both look bigger than Zest, which is 5 ounces. Dove and Phase III have a cardboard inner wrapper which makes them look bigger than they are. Among the ordinary or "soap" soaps, you also have such cute dilemmas as trying to compare the value of a "medium-size" 5½-ounce bar of Ivory with a "medium" 5-ounce bar of Camay Beauty Soap, which is almost as difficult as figuring which makes you more beautiful.

The actual contents of aerosol hair sprays is especially mystifying to consumers, and has been compounded by the proliferation of sizes. Malcolm Jensen, U.S. Bureau of Standards official, warned toiletries manufacturers late in 1969 that the Commerce Department might have to act to reduce the multiplicity of sizes if the industry itself did not. Virginia Knauer pointed out that there are almost three dozen quantity-sizes of hair sprays, including such value riddles as 12.5-, 13.5- and 13.7-ounce sizes.

Moreover, the propellant is part of the product content. One manufacturer may put 4 ounces of propellant into a 14-ounce can. Another packager, making the same kind of product, may use 8 ounces of a less expensive propellant in a 14-ounce can, Mrs. Knauer observed. The buyer thinks she gets 14 ounces of "product" in either can. Does she? Under present circumstances, only her manufacturer knows for sure.

As a result of such comparison problems, Bess Myerson Grant, New York City's Consumer Commissioner, reports that a survey by her department found that even experienced shoppers fail to select the best buys as much as 40 percent of the time. This failure, Mrs. Grant warns, may cost you up to 11 cents of every food shopping dollar.

Consumers have this needless and wasteful problem because Congress failed to require standard sizes, as the original Senate Truth-in-Packaging bill called for.

Instead, Congress authorized the Secretary of Commerce to determine whether reasonably comparable products are being sold in an undue proliferation of package sizes which impairs consumers' ability to compare value. If the Secretary finds such undue proliferation, he must ask the packagers to develop a voluntary standard for package sizes, presumably to end this undue proliferation. If, after a year, he finds that no standard has been established, he must recommend to Congress whether it should enact regulatory authority to deal with the problem.

The Secretary delegated this responsibility to the National Bureau of Standards. To carry it out, the bureau has eliminated those categories of products whose net contents are specified by state law (milk, bread) and those sold in random packages, such as meat, cheese and fresh produce. (The elimination of bread has been an especially harmful decision because of the proliferation of sizes, even under some state laws, and the random and odd weights noted in Chapter 8.)

Then the bureau asks a weights and measures agency (state or local) in each of the eight census regions to report the package sizes for each other category of products found in a large shopping center supermarket and in a rural supermarket. On the basis of this sixteen-store survey, the bureau makes an administrative judgment as to whether undue proliferation exists in a particular product line.

In March, 1970, the department told Congress that in its judgment 176 categories of commodities offered no undue proliferation. These include such products as coffee, which does come in standard-sized packages, and those such as baking powder, sold in few sizes and thus presenting no severe problem in comparing values.

So far, the bureau has not determined that undue proliferation does or does not exist. Rather, on the basis of the sixteen-store survey and its administrative judgment, the bureau has adopted the method of deciding whether to call producers together, if that seems necessary in a particular product line, and to urge them to reduce the number of sizes in which they offer products. So far, no group of producers has refused to meet to discuss reducing the number of package sizes, if requested, or to establish a voluntary products standards committee to that end. For example, packagers agreed to reduce the number of salad oil container sizes from 15 to 7; of instant coffee, from 10 to 8; of peanut butter, from 30 to 12; of detergent package sizes from 24 to 6; of jellies and preserves, from 16 to 10; of candy, from 153 to 72; of cookies and crackers, from 73 to 56.

Along similar lines, packagers of dry cereals agreed to package in whole ounces only (except for individual-portion boxes) and reduce the number of sizes from thirty-three to sixteen. Frozen vegetable packers agreed to eliminate fractional ounces, but managed not to agree to reduce their thirteen package sizes. The manufacturers of paper towels reduced their jungle of different sizes, plies and dimensions from thirty-three to eight, and also now state on the label the square feet per package.

The bureau also found mouthwashes offered in twenty-nine different package sizes. Under its prodding, producers agreed to cut these to eleven.

By the time the Commerce Department reported to Congress

in 1970, it had encouraged packagers of thirty different product categories to reduce the proliferation of packages. Also, packagers of five different product categories did initiate a voluntary product standards procedure.

But on the whole, the reductions made so far in the confusing and costly number of packages have been small in comparison to the dimensions of this money-wasting problem for consumers and for the stores.

For example, David Angevine notes that packagers of mayonnaise and salad dressing agreed to reduce the number of sizes from five to four. Later, they told the bureau they wanted to add a fifth—48 ounces. So they are now back where they were.

Under the potato chip simplified-size program, packagers still may offer fifty-three different quantities up to 4 pounds. While the bureau has made no determination that this still constitutes undue proliferation, it did continue to pressure the Potato Chip Institute. In three regions (mostly in the East), producer members then accepted a tougher standard that would permit a maximum of seven quantities. Then negotiations blew sky-high when the Justice Department indicted a group of West Coast potato chip processors for conspiring to fix prices and restrain competition, and in its catch-all bill of particulars, charged that the processors had met to agree on package size.

Instant tea packagers, after agreeing on a simplified quantity pattern involving ounces per package, asked the bureau to shift to a per-cup yield, and the bureau agreed.

A major block to solving the packaging problem has been the meager appropriations provided by Congress to do the job. To administer sections 5 and 9 of the act and voluntary product standards, the bureau spent $130,000 in fiscal 1968, $208,000 in 1969, $155,000 in 1970 and expected to spend $149,000 in 1971.

Malcolm Jensen and Eric Vadelund, bureau officials working on the program, told Angevine they had no way to measure industries' reaction. At meetings, some packagers have volunteered comments that the bureau's efforts have created no difficulties. Others have said the effort to reduce the number of package sizes has enabled them to improve their inventory controls. A few small packagers have told Vadelund that since they are less able to introduce new packages than their larger competitors, the bureau's efforts have tended to equalize competition.

At the March, 1970, hearing, Senator Frank Moss, chairman of the Senate Consumer Subcommittee, criticized the department's extra-legal approach to package proliferation, and the department defended it. Clearly, Congress intended that the department should determine for each category of commodities whether there was or was not undue proliferation of packaging. The department has made no such determination—not for any category. It has simply exercised its administrative judgment, Angevine observes.

Formal determination of undue proliferation admittedly is a time-consuming process. The bureau would have needed (1) far more evidence than the skimpy sixteen-store survey provides; (2) a formal proposal of determination in the *Federal Register;* (3) a sixty-day opportunity for producers and others to comment; (4) perhaps a revised proposal in light of these comments that would again be published, and again be open to written comments; (5) a public hearing; (6) the determination, reflecting both the comments and the hearing.

Then if the department found undue proliferation—and the courts upheld the finding—the department would ask the packagers to develop a voluntary product standard. A year later, if they had not done so or had adopted a standard and were not observing it, the department would report to Congress and recommend whether it should enact regulatory legislation.

While this is a long process, it gives consumers an opportunity to participate in the determination of undue proliferation. As it is, under the bureau's extra-legal approach, consumers have no opportunity formally to challenge its administrative judgment of what is due or undue proliferation, which products should receive attention next and whether the simplified quantity patterns represent any or sufficient improvement. The bureau can put a commodity on its "undue proliferation" list one week, move it off the next week, and back the following week.

For consumers, the bureau's approach is like gathering clouds, Angevine comments. The act mentions "adequate manufacturer, packer, distributor, and consumer repre-

sentation," but this relates only to "procedures for the development of voluntary products standards" under an earlier law.

For whatever reason, neither President Johnson nor President
Nixon asked Congress for funds for determining whether there is
undue proliferation of sizes. Not being asked, Congress did not
provide.

The problem is whether the bureau should use formal
determination processes, knowing it can sequester only enough
funds from other programs to touch a few commodities each
year. Or should it exercise its own informal judgment about
which groups of packagers to call together, and see what it could
get them to do quite voluntarily?

In Angevine's judgment, the bureau has reduced package
proliferation to a level that perhaps forestalls serious consumer
revolt, yet that continues to impair the reasonable ability of
consumers to make value comparisons. As the hearing record
showed, the Commerce Department feels it has handled—or
should not touch—products representing 88 percent of
consumers' expenditures. It feels its job is almost done—except
for some record-keeping when the mayonnaise people want to
add a 3-pound jar. It would much rather switch the conversation
to unit pricing.

The department has not asked any group of producers to
simplify package proliferation by adopting a voluntary product
standard. The five groups that voluntarily did so are the
packagers of green olives, instant nonfat dry milk, instant
potatoes, school paste and toothpaste.

With the Truth-in-Packaging law providing only limited help,
the more aware consumers more recently have tried to convince
retailers to post the price per pound, quart or pint, as well as the
price per package. This is called "unit pricing," or, in the
grocery trade, "dual pricing." Legislation also has been
introduced in Congress and in several states and cities to that
end. Massachusetts in 1970 became the first state to pass state-
wide enabling legislation.

Under unit pricing, stores would have to label canned tuna
fish, for example, as "6 ½ ounces, 37 cents; 91 cents a pound."
In most areas stores do this for store-wrapped meats, poultry,
fish, cheese and some produce, and there is no reason why they

cannot for packaged and canned foods. It is illogical, and perplexing to the consumer, to sell fresh meat, poultry and fish by the pound, but canned or, often, frozen versions by the package.

If this responsibility is put on the stores, it is reasonable to expect that they in turn will press canners, packers and bakers to use more uniform and standard sizes. Eventually both stores and manufacturers would benefit as well as consumers.

Of course, if Congress had passed that part of the original Truth-in-Packaging proposal seeking uniform weights and measures for packaged products (pints, quarts, pounds, half-pounds), the present drive for unit pricing would not be necessary.

Already by 1971 some consumers around the country are beginning to see the difference in real prices of many packaged foods as some stores voluntarily adopt unit pricing. Consumers can see, for example, that the size, brand and type can make a difference of virtually 100 percent and sometimes more in the true cost of many staples.

If you know the price per unit, you can more readily compare values and select the item offering best value for your particular cooking purpose.

For example, you can see the difference in cost among (1) different brands, (2) different sizes and (3) different versions of the same food. You could pay as much as 56 cents a pint or more for mayonnaise in half-pint jars under the national brand names or you could buy the store's own brand, and pay as little as 33 cents a pint in the pint size. That saving is achieved by buying both the private brand *and* the larger size. You could save even further by using salad dressing instead, and pay as little as 20 cents.

Unit pricing, or your own calculations if stores in your area do not yet do it, also would show some revealing pricing maneuvers by the manufacturers. For example, you may find some brands of salad dressing selling for the same price as the same manufacturer's mayonnaise, even though salad dressings generally are less expensive.

Unit pricing also helps you keep track of concealed price increases sometimes effected by food and toiletries manufacturers. Instead of increasing the price itself when they want to raise the price, manufacturers may keep the same price but reduce the contents. The House of Representatives Consumer Subcommittee compiled a list of over six hundred products that had been reduced in quantity from 1964 to 1968. This committee and other observers reported examples of such reductions as 7 ½ ounces to 6 ½ for canned peanuts, and 12 ½ to 11 ½ for a brand-name shampoo.

Greatest price differences revealed by unit pricing are between stores' own brands and national brands. But there also are differences among the national brands, too, as the comparative prices of tomato juices and tuna fish show.

The price differences between smallest and largest sizes also are striking. The differences between medium and largest sizes are less drastic, but still important.

Many consumer co-ops and a number of supermarket chains also have adopted or are experimenting with unit pricing. When Esther Peterson, the first presidential consumer advisor, served in 1970 as consumer consultant to the Giant Food Stores in Washington, one of her first tasks was supervising the introduction of unit pricing by the pound, quart, count and square feet (for paper and foil). She pointed out to consumers that they cannot, of course, tell the quality of products by looking at the price per pound but they can tell how much their preferences are costing them.

An effort by Commissioner Bess Myerson Grant to require unit pricing on six specific foods, including bread and cereals, was stopped when the New York State Food Merchants Association went to court. The judge agreed that unit pricing would help consumers, but said the commissioner had exceeded her authority. At this writing a bill has been introduced into the City Council there to provide that authority.

Cost is not a factor, Seymour Klanfer, vice-president of the New York City Federation of Cooperatives, told me. He finds that there is not enough extra cost to pass on to the consumer. Too, where educational campaigns have been coordinated with the introduction of unit pricing, consumers generally do understand and use it.

Similarly, the president of the Benner Tea Co. Stores in Iowa reported that the availability of computers has made unit pricing feasible at less than $100 a year per store for maintenance expense. The Star store in Rhode Island, after adopting unit pricing in cooperation with that state's Consumer Council, reported that there is no extra cost to the consumer when computations are done by computer.

Even the New York State Food Merchants Association, after it had halted by court action the New York City unit-pricing program, changed its mind. It said it would not oppose what it called "realistic" state legislation which would eliminate, as in Massachusetts, smaller stores from such requirements.

Where the unit prices have been easy to see and understand, as when stores have put them on shelf signs, consumers have found them most helpful. But when stores have grouped unit prices, as in one big chart for 103 different sizes, brands and types of cereals, or in price sheets at the end of the aisle, they themselves have made the unit prices hard to use.

Grocery trade associations have tended to hide their opposition behind avowed concern for the small grocer. Actually, unit pricing would be easiest for him. Many of the foods he sells already are priced by the pound or quart: milk, cheese, eggs, much of the produce, meat, fish, coffees, many of the baked goods, luncheon meats and delicatessen items, ice cream and so on. The small grocer does not carry the great variety of dry groceries found in large supermarkets. Too, the small store changes prices less often than do large ones. For certain items with preprinted prices such as bread and baked goods, the supplier would have to preprint the unit price.

If your own local stores do not yet provide unit pricing, the potential savings are big enough to make it worthwhile to do this much calculating yourself. It is a nuisance. But once you have the better buys picked out, you won't have to spend much time at it.

EXAMPLES OF COMPARATIVE COSTS SHOWN BY UNIT PRICING*

	Item Size	Item Price	Cost per Measure
Tomato Juice			
Star's Own Food Club	18 oz.	16¢	28¢ quart
Campbell's	17½	18	33
Star's Own Food Club	46	33	23
Libby's	46	35	24
Campbell's	46	37	26
Glorietta California	46	42	29
Star's Own Food Club	5½	6/49	48
Libby's	5½	6/57	55
Sacramento California	5½	6/57	55
Tuna Fish, Grated			
Co-op, light, in oil	6 oz.	29¢	77¢ pound
Tuna Fish, Chunk			
Co-op, light, in oil	9½ oz.	43¢	74¢ pound
Co-op, light, in oil	6½	31	76
White Star, light, in oil	6½	37	91
White Star, light, in oil	9¼	55	95
Starkist, light, in oil	9¼	56	97
White Star, light, in oil	3¼	25	$1.23
White Star, white, in oil	6½	45	$1.11
Tuna Fish, Solid			
Co-op, light, in oil	7 oz.	38¢	87¢ pound
White Star, light, in oil	7	45	$1.03
Co-op, white, in oil	7	41	94
Co-op, light, in brine	7	34	78
Co-op, white, in brine	7	45	$1.03
Starkist, white, in water	7	46	$1.05

*Tomato juice prices from Star stores, Rhode Island; tuna prices from Berkeley, California, co-ops. Prices will vary at different times.

12

WHY CONSUMERS WANT TO KNOW THE "PULL DATES"

Food has become too expensive to buy and throw out. In an age of many prepackaged foods, that often is what people have had to do. Such problems as packaged cold cuts that soon become slimy in the home refrigerator, thawed and refrozen vegetable packages, milk about to turn sour and stale cheese all have become a serious controversy.

That is why a national demand has developed for "open dating" of perishable foods. Most prepackaged foods already have "pull dates," beyond which they are not supposed to be sold. But the dates are in code numbers, which vary from store to store and often from product to product, and also often are changed. They are the little numbers you notice on bread wrappers, milk cartons (in areas where open dates are not required), and on egg cartons and meat packages.

Finding out what dates these numbers or letters represent has become a game of espionage often even harder than breaking the Japanese intelligence code in World War II.

The irritation over stale or souring foods, which can get quite emotional, has been so widespread that in 1970, some sixty congressmen had joined together in bipartisan sponsorship of a bill to require foods to be marked openly with the last day they are palatable and safe.

As this is written, the bill has not been enacted. Some con-

sumer co-ops and at least one large chain, Safeway, voluntarily are showing the pull dates, or the less frequent "push
dates" (the dates of packing). In Chicago, Jewel and National
Tea Company stores both announced they would make available information on the codes used in their stores. The Berkeley co-op supermarkets published their codes in their *Co-op
News*. A number of other stores provide code books for shoppers to use if they wish.

Some supermarkets defend their secrecy by arguing that
consumers would buy only the latest packages. The stores would
be stuck with the older goods and prices would be raised to cover
these losses.

But consumers pay for the spoiled foods either way. Moreover, costs can be restrained by proper rotation and can even
be reduced rather than raised if open dating encourages stores
to be more careful about amounts prepackaged, as in the
case of cold cuts and other meats, or left in stores by route
salesmen, as in the case of milk, bread and cake.

In fact, open dates even would make it easier for clerks to
rotate stock properly and to know when to pull out-of-date
foods, Helen Black, Berkeley home economist, has pointed out.
At home, too, you would know which items are oldest and
should be used first.

The stores also pointed out that consumers can return spoiled
foods. But Ellis Levin, assistant to then-congressman, Leonard
Farbstein, observed that they often are afraid or embarrassed
to do so.

Pending legislation or more widespread voluntary revelation
by stores, you can protect yourself to a limited extent by learning
some of the codes used in local stores. Sometimes a store
manager or clerk will tell you what some of the code numbers
represent, although some are afraid to, and some are not
certain themselves what dates the codes represent.

Bread is usually coded by the color of the tie on the end of the
wrapper. In Detroit, Trudy Lieberman, *Free Press* consumer
reporter, found that in one store red indicated the bread was
brought in on Monday, white was for Tuesday, yellow for
Thursday, orange for Friday and green for Saturday. Other
bakers used different color ties or number codes. For example,

she found three brands coded A19, 1902 and 192 and concluded that this meant the loaves should be out of the store by the nineteenth of the month.

Miss Lieberman found bacon coded 0192, meaning it should be out by February 19; 2100, meaning a pull date of February 10; and 213, indicating February 13. Meats were coded with letters, NW meaning packaged on Wednesday.

A&P stores in several cities use a letter and a numeral for meat coding, with the numeral representing the date of the week: 1 for Monday, and so on. Apparently this is the big chain's national practice, at least as this is written.

Other chains have been found to use four-digit or two-letter codes. In Cleveland, *Plain Dealer* reporter Douglas Bloomfield found Kroger using a letter and numeral code, with the numeral indicating the week the item was packed and the letter the day: M for Monday, and so on.

The American Meat Institute's code is used for meat by a number of chains. In this code the first and last numbers indicate the month and the middle numbers indicate the day of the month.

For coffee, some stores used a code embossed in the cover or bottom of the can, with the letters A to L for the month, followed by one numeral for the year. But here, too, codes vary.

The codes on eggs vary, but often are relatively clear. They have such expiration symbols as 023, meaning October 23, or simply 23, meaning the twenty-third day of the current month.

Whether milk should be dated or not has been a controversy for many years. Fresh milk will last in a home refrigerator at least a week. But if it is already several days old, it may not. In cities where milk does not have an open date, the code number usually can be found either printed or embossed on the top flap (on the bottom for cottage cheese and yogurt). The number indicates the expiration day.

At present, only in six areas is open dating required for milk: New York City, Baltimore, St. Louis, Birmingham, suburban Philadelphia and New Jersey, the *USDA Farm Index* reports.

13

THE SALMONELLA PROBLEM
IN PROCESSED FOODS

Just because food comes in a clean-looking package or cellophane wrapping, you cannot take for granted that it is really "clean." The widespread occurrence of salmonella infection, a form of food poisoning, has been traced at least in part to the increasing use of so-called "convenience" foods requiring little or no heating at home.

Ironically, one of the justifications claimed by the food industry and U.S. Agriculture Department spokesmen for processed foods with their extra cost is their "cleanliness" in contrast to the mythical "open cracker barrel" of old-time grocery stores.

But it turns out that cellophane can hide a multitude of organisms. You know whether or not your hands and kitchen are clean when you prepare food. You do not know the sanitary conditions in a specific food factory at a specific time.

The facts are that over 2,000,000 people get sick each year from contaminated food, and the chief culprit is the salmonella organism. Other estimates of intestinal illness have ranged as high as 10,000,000 a year. Food poisoning is second only to colds as the most frequent cause of illness, government authorities say.

In many cases of healthy adults, salmonella produces only a twenty-four hour diarrhea. In the past and even now, relatively few cases have been diagnosed as salmonella, largely because public health authorities did not realize until the late 1960's the full extent of this form of contamination. But in infants and elderly people salmonella infection can be serious and even dangerous.

Dr. Ernest Ager of the Washington State Health Department has called the salmonella problem "a national disgrace." Now that the extent of the problem is realized, the FDA and the U.S. Public Health Service are trying, rather desperately and anxiously with their limited funds and personnel, to control it. In 1969, FDA inaugurated a national center for microbiological analysis of food products.

In some cases industry has cooperated in the government's campaign. But in some cases, such as that of suppliers of animal by-products used in animal feed (which can start the chain of contamination), industry apparently has been unconcerned.

In the late 1960's and 1970 there have had to be recalls of widely sold packaged products, including dried milk and products such as commercially sold custard pies and chocolate candy. Dried milk and dried, liquid or frozen eggs used widely by commercial bakers and other food factories often are implicated in outbreaks of salmonella.

One of the reasons for the increased concern is that food no longer is sold primarily locally. Factories nowadays ship food products all over the country, with the resultant possibility of nationwide outbreaks of food poisoning.

Another problem is that once the salmonella organism gets into food-manufacturing machinery it is hard to eradicate.

Frozen prepared foods, the so-called "heat-and-serve" items, appear to be a particular problem. They are especially susceptible to microbiological contamination, reports Charles C. Johnson, Jr., a Public Health Service administrator. Furthermore, Johnson says, "We are actually doing very little in the way of standards to assure their safety."

With frozen precooked foods thawing and refreezing, as sometimes occurs in the distribution chain, these foods can be more dangerous than uncooked frozen foods, such as frozen vegetables. Precooked foods in general are more subject to contamination before freezing than the simpler frozen foods. They contain a number of ingredients, take longer in preparation and also sometimes require more handling in the factory, the U.S. Agriculture Department has pointed out.

For example, the gravy for a frozen precooked dinner may be prepared before the potatoes are ready, and thus the danger of contamination is increased. Or some preparation may require hand operations, such as the boning of chicken, which also can increase contamination risks.

The Agriculture Department points out that those dangers of contamination are further multiplied because frozen precooked foods often are merely warmed, not really cooked, before being served in the home. So frozen precooked foods especially need to be handled with care, making sure to avoid letting them thaw on the way home and keeping them frozen so that any bacteria cannot multiply.

One of the difficulties in guarding against contamination is that ready-to-eat foods are not usually subject to high cooking heats before they are served at home. They may be merely warmed a little, or even not at all. High heat does help to control harmful bacteria.

In some cases manufacturers have had to institute nationwide recalls for such products as candy bars and dried noodle soups, or more quietly go about buying up the stock from stores. Some factories even had to close down to try to eradicate salmonella infection from their plants, as in the case of an eastern factory which made frozen desserts. These were used in catered affairs in a number of states. In just one week in April, 1967, outbreaks involving two thousand to three thousand people occurred at catered affairs in New York City, which served these commercially prepared desserts. The contamination finally was traced to the use of nonpasteurized sugared egg yolks.

There also are growing problems associated with the new infant food formulations, many of them using dried milk.

Salmonella infection could be greatly reduced if the safety of frozen eggs, widely used commercially, could be assured, Johnson says. New York City, for example, now requires thorough pasteurization by local processors of such "broken out" eggs.

But such local control is not enough in an era when processed foods are shipped all over the country. Nationwide regulation of egg products really is needed and would be required by legislation under consideration in Congress as this is written.

Only eight states presently require pasteurization of egg products, Congressman Graham Purcell of Texas has pointed out (Colorado, California, Georgia, Minnesota, Oregon, South Dakota, Utah, Wisconsin).

Passage of this bill, together with intensified efforts by FDA, which already have helped control salmonella contamination of dried milk, would be a vital first step. At that, full control of the salmonella problem apparently will take at least until the late 1970's.

But while government intervention to require high sanitation standards in food and feed factories is of first importance, care also is needed in the home.

As one safeguard, make sure that any nonfat dry milk you buy carries the U.S. Extra grade mark in a shield on the package. The grade mark not only assures good flavor and instant solubility, but that the product was made in a government-inspected sanitary plant.

Salmonella bacteria are killed by heat, so that normally cooked meat and poultry offer no risk, according to the USDA. The department does, however, advise serving food soon after cooking. If not, refrigerate promptly. You really do not have to wait for cooked foods to cool off completely before refrigerating. Food may not be safe to eat if held for more than three or four hours at room temperatures, including preparation and serving time.

In addition to general kitchen sanitation and personal hygiene, the department also advises keeping hot foods *hot* (above 140 degrees).

The Consumers' Association of Canada, which also has investigated the salmonella problem, warns that it is important to clean up right away after preparing poultry. Chopping boards and knives must be scrupulously cleaned before being used for other foods. Packages and wrappings which have contained uncooked poultry should be put in a bag or rolled up in a newspaper before being put in the garbage can.

SECTION

II

BUYING THE MOST FOR $100,000

14.

ARE YOU YOUR OWN WORST ENEMY IN BUYING FOOD?

Shopping for best food values is difficult enough these days when a supermarket may have as many as 8,000-10,000 items, and many foods come prepackaged with inadequate information on what they contain, and are presold by mass TV advertising.

But often housewives are their own worst enemies. They whisk through the supermarkets, typically spending in seventeen minutes the $15 their husbands typically work four hours to earn. They fail to study the ingredients shown on the package, or to calculate the cost per pound of the many competing products and brands.

One USDA survey found that fewer than seven out of ten shoppers even looked at grades before buying eggs. Only one out of ten looked for the grade in buying butter, turkeys or milk. If you want to know something else, fewer than half even checked the prices.

Many did at least look at labels of packaged foods before they bought, but 20 to 36 percent said they did not, or looked only long enough to know what it was they were buying.

Another survey, in 1970, by Gallup for the American Newspaper Publishers Association, found that four out of ten shoppers usually make price comparisons before they go shopping. But the other side of that coin is that six out of ten do not. The ones that do usually shop more than one market, have a weekly food bill between $21 and $30, save both newspaper and direct mail ads and come from larger families, *Supermarket News* reported.

A Michigan survey found that nearly a fourth of the homemakers questioned shop by trial and error. Another fourth buy whatever they want without regard to cost. When they get home, only about half are satisfied with their selections, and feel they have done a good job.

Women perform this way nowadays not because they are lazy but because shopping has become more difficult, even a grim affair of trying to find values among the crowded shelves or shopping at several stores for their specials.

But trying to get through with shopping quickly, instead of treating it as seriously and professionally as earning a living, makes you a target for manipulation. Shopping can be interesting, if not really "fun," if you treat it as a skill.

One problem is that in an age of heavy advertising and prepackaged foods, many women have lost confidence in their own judgment. They tend to rely on a well-known name or to assume that a higher price means better quality.

A number of tests have shown that sometimes the same item priced a little higher sold even better. One such test several years ago found that leaner pork butts and hams, called "meat-type" pork, sold better if they were priced six cents higher than if only two cents higher than regular pork.

There is a good deal of evidence—both empirical and statistical—that today's young housewife is likely to be nutritionally uninformed and often a casual, even complaisant, shopper for her family's food needs—complaisant because she lives in an age of processed foods often promoted as "fortified," "enriched," and so on, and she may be leaving the nutritional task to the manufacturers, and trusting the government. But financially, as this book should show, she should not be so trusting.

Women of the older generation at least were subjected, during the war years, to the Red Cross classes and constant nutritional advice and guidance in waste prevention from government agencies and community organizations. There no longer is this kind of widespread program.

But one of the most important causes for haphazard shopping

and unknowing use of pseudo-convenience items is the rationalization that only pennies are involved. Look at it this way. If you have a family, you probably spend $2,000 a year for food, perhaps $100,000 in your family's lifetime.

In an era of self-service shopping, women who do not use what information is available to them for selecting best buys even can be led to buy a particular brand just by a picture on a package or even its color.

For example, merely putting the picture of a spoon on the Betty Crocker cake mix package helped to make that brand the leading seller, Louis Cheskin, one of the most successful "motivational researchers," revealed in *Secrets of Marketing Success*.

Putting Parliament cigarettes in a blue package increased their sales. In fact, the researchers found that when the package had a linen finish, 80 percent of the smokers tested thought the cigarettes tasted finer, Cheskin reported. Even just putting an illustration of a crest on the package boosted sales of Marlboro cigarettes.

Cheskin says that the choices people make are not motivated by logic "but we seek rational reasons for making them." According to him, we think we are buying useful quality, but actually we are attracted by the styling. Sometimes we are aware of this, but we cover up—"we try to make ourselves appear rational."

Thus, over twice as many housewives in a test considered Gold Imperial Margarine in one package to be "higher priced" than in another package.

Cheskin did not mention this, but it has become obvious that much of a mother's buying now is dominated by children who in turn are dominated by television. This kind of forced buying is especially noticeable nowadays among such products as cereals, soft drinks, and the milkshake products sold with musical shakers.

There is even less reason for women to be manipulated by the color and design of a package than by their children. All they need do is take the time to read the lists of ingredients and net weights to see, at least approximately, what one brand actually provides, compared with another.

A DuPont study found that the average supermarketing

shopper makes about half of her purchases on an unplanned or impulse basis. Most often the unplanned purchases are convenience foods, such as frozen dinners; snack foods, such as marshmallows; or ancillary cleaning products, such as sponges or sponge cloths, John Crichton noted in a 1966 address to the American Association of Advertising Agencies.

Not only manufacturers, but also the supermarkets manipulate customers, Anastasio warns. One of the favorite selling tricks is to feature an advertised special on coffee with a big display at the end of an aisle, and next to it a display of cheap candy. The store gets a 50 percent margin on the candy.

Much of supermarket selling today relies on such impulse buying. Displays of high-point items at aisle ends and the checkout counter often are aimed especially at children, Anastasio points out. The mothers, on the other hand, are manipulated into buying expensive foods, such as frozen vegetables with a little butter sauce, by the display of these next to the cheaper ordinary vegetables without the added butter.

The Berkeley Cooperative uses many store exhibits "to goad people" into reading labels. "When you ask them to guess which bottle contains more soda, and they guess wrong, they realize that the label is worth watching," Betsy Wood reports.

It is never enough merely to glance at the face of the package, and take for granted either the relative amount of content or the ingredients. There are many variations of size, and indication of weight, in soaps all called "bath size." Different packages of frozen vegetables may contain 8, 9 or 10 ounces, but seem to be the same size as they lie in the store's freezer cabinet. The faces of the packages actually are much the same size. But the thicknesses vary. That also is why a product such as Shake'n Bake, with only 2 $\frac{3}{8}$ ounces of content, looks as big on the store shelf as the box of Nabisco cracker meal, with 9 ½ ounces.

Another apparent reason for the failure of many women to learn to buy with real skill is that they tend to rely on the government more than they truly can. That same USDA survey [14] found most of the women believed a number of foods are government-graded which are not so graded—bacon, for example. T.Q. Hutchinson, USDA economist, interpreted this "halo effect" as arising from an assumption by consumers that since some meats are graded, all are. Several women even asked, "Aren't all foods graded by the government?"

The answer, unfortunately both for consumers and the general state of the economy, is no, they are not. A list of some that are is provided in Chapter 17.

Finding Best Values

Earlier chapters of this book have pointed out many of the better food values. Following is a summary of a number of knowledgeable practices that can help you defend your family against today's cynical, wasteful food merchandising, processing and promotion practices by large food corporations. These are the techniques that can make every dollar you spend bring as much genuine food value as is possible in the present circumstances of inadequate standards and fearful administration of them. Succeeding chapters in this section provide additional information on a number of the most important techniques: buying by grade, the use of private brands, shopping specials and planning food budgets. The table at the end of this chapter shows you how a knowing shopper can buy a $27 market basket of food for $17 by using these methods:

1. Don't let the advertising and merchandising gunslingers persuade you or your family to buy foods you do not really need or that are not suitable or offer only pseudo-convenience at an exaggerated price. Buy on the basis of your own needs and with as close examination as possible. For any food you need to buy, you can form your own judgments.

2. Give the same time and care to food planning and buying as to other important jobs—as much as to, say, making a dress or working for money outside your home. Surveys have shown that the typical shopper buys thirty-two items from fifty locations in about fifteen minutes of shopping time. That's an average of one purchase every twenty-eight seconds—obviously only time enough to walk over and look at the name of the product and perhaps the price.

3. Read the list of ingredients on the package to know what you are buying and which product is least expensive for similar ingredients. Especially read the ingredients list of *new* products, and double-especially if they are advertised heavily on TV.

4. As emphasized in this book, beware the pseudo-convenience of many of today's ready-to-eat foods. Because an advertising man says, "This is more convenient!" you don't have to respond like a TV-trained automaton and echo in your head, "This is more convenient!"

5. Buy the grade best suited to your cooking purposes. Usually there are two or three grades or qualities for the same product, as explained in Chapter 17.

6. We have been conditioned to buy everything under an advertised brand name. But the unadvertised brands of canned goods and other groceries and the so-called private brands of the large retailers offer significant savings, as reported in Chapter 16.

7. Check the number of ounces on the container, even though various brands on the shelf or in the frozen-foods cabinets seem to be the same size. The assumption by manufacturers is that most housewives are poor at arithmetic and do not want to make the necessary comparisons of weights.

In cleaning supplies, too, you need to compare the weights, and in paper goods the actual square inches provided must be stated, under the Truth-in-Packaging law. For example, you may find the biggest-selling brand of ammonia, Parson's, has 28 ounces, while some supermarket private brands are a full quart (32 ounces). At 27 cents a bottle, the brand-name product costs 31 cents a quart, compared with as little as 19 cents for a private brand—Co-op, in this case. (At that, Anastasio reports the Co-op Ammonia tests 6.12 percent ammonia while the name brand tests only 3.3 percent.)

8. Buy the larger sizes, as explained in Chapter 18.

9. Plan your meals around the advertised specials. As shown in Chapter 15, the savings from knowledgeable sale shopping can be important.

10. Buy standard foods rather than higher-cost versions with added ingredients—for example, standard white, rye or whole-wheat breads instead of rolls or special breads, basic cereals rather than those with added ingredients, plain cheeses, standard milk instead of milk with additional fortification if sold at a higher price, standard rice, noodles and so on.

11. Buy medium-sized fruit and vegetables, rather than the specially selected perfect-looking large ones.

12. Especially watch spending for meat and commercial baked goods. Meat is your single largest expense. If you can keep spending for meat, poultry and fish under 25 percent of your total food expenses most months, you are managing well.

Because of meat's steadily rising cost and its effect on your food expenses, even your whole budget, at the end of this chapter we have provided tables of comparative protein costs (that is what you really buy), and costs per serving at early 1971 prices. There also is a chart for calculating costs per serving as prices change.

HOW TO BUY $27 WORTH OF FOOD FOR $17

Item	Typical Price	Savings Method Used	Price Paid*
7 loaves bread	$2.10	Private brand, largest size	$1.40
6 qts. milk	1.80	Private brand, gallon size	1.58
1½ lb. nonfat milk	1.15	Private brand, larger size	.79
4 6-oz. frozen orange juice	.99	Private brand, 8-oz. size	.68
1 46-oz. tomato juice	.41	Private brand on sale	.33
4 oz. instant coffee	.89	Private brand, 6-oz. size	.65
2 10-oz. frozen mixed vegetables	.53	Private brand, 2-lb. cello. bag	.17
1 8-oz. frozen peas, cream sauce	.37	2-lb. pour bag, home sauce	.19
2 12-oz. corn flakes	.70	Private brand, 18-oz. size	.27
1 box round crackers	.38	Private brand	.29
1 lb. spaghetti	.27	Private brand on sale	.20
2 cans canned hash	1.08	Private brand on sale	.86
1 pkg. instant flavored oatmeal	.43	One-minute oatmeal	.11
2 cans tuna	1.02	Grated or flake type, private brand	.66
2 boxes coating mix	.54	Substitute cracker meal, eggs, fat	.31

Item	Price	Note	Adjusted
4 frozen pot pies	1.16	Private brand, weekend special	.76
2 frozen franks/beans dinners	.82	Substitute cooked franks, canned beans, applesauce	.35
1 lb. margarine	.38	Private brand	.23
1 lb. American cheese	1.04	2-lb. loaf instead of slices	.82
½ lb. flavored cottage cheese	.28	Private brand, larger size, home flavored	.20
1 honeydew melon	.69	Weekend special	.49
1 head lettuce	.37	Cabbage for cole slaw	.15
2 boxes facial tissues	.70	Private brand on sale	.39
1 bottle dishwashing detergent	.59	Private brand, larger size	.29
1 jar noodles and chicken	.50	Dried noodles, boned chicken	.21
1 lb. bologna	1.15	Chunk instead of sliced	.69
4 lbs. broiler parts	2.60	Weekend special on whole chicken	1.45
3 lbs. chuck steak	2.25	Weekend special	1.59
2 lbs. pork loin roast	2.19	Substitute pork shoulder on sale	1.10
Total $27.38			Total $17.21

*As of early 1971; prices adjusted for same quantity where necessary.

COST OF FOOD AT HOME AT THREE LEVELS*

	Cost for 1 week			Cost for 1 month		
	Low-cost plan	Moderate-cost plan	Liberal plan	Low-cost plan	Moderate-cost plan	Liberal plan
FAMILIES						
Family of 2:						
20 to 35 years**	$18.50	$23.40	$28.80	$80.10	$102.00	$124.70
55 to 75 years**	15.30	19.60	23.50	65.70	85.20	102.10
Family of 4:						
Preschool children	26.80	34.00	41.40	116.30	148.20	179.80
School children	31.10	39.70	49.80	134.90	172.60	211.20
INDIVIDUALS						
Children, under 1 year	3.60	4.50	5.00	15.70	19.70	22.00
1 to 3 years	4.50	5.80	6.90	19.90	25.00	30.00
3 to 6 years	5.40	7.00	8.40	23.60	30.40	36.40
6 to 9 years	6.70	8.50	10.60	28.70	36.90	45.90

Girls, 9 to 12 years	7.60	9.70	11.40	32.60	42.20	49.30
12 to 15 years	8.30	10.80	13.00	36.00	46.80	56.50
15 to 20 years	8.50	10.70	12.70	36.80	46.50	55.10
Boys, 9 to 12 years	7.70	9.90	12.00	33.40	43.00	51.90
12 to 15 years	9.00	11.80	14.10	39.10	51.40	61.10
15 to 20 years	10.40	13.20	16.00	45.00	57.20	69.00
Women, 20 to 35 years	7.80	9.90	11.90	33.80	43.10	51.70
35 to 55 years	7.50	9.60	11.50	32.50	41.50	49.80
55 to 75 years	6.40	8.20	9.80	27.50	35.60	42.40
Pregnant	9.30	11.60	13.60	40.20	50.20	59.30
Men, 20 to 35 years	9.00	11.40	14.20	39.00	49.60	61.70
35 to 55 years	8.40	10.60	13.00	36.20	46.20	56.30
55 to 75 years	7.50	9.60	11.60	32.20	41.80	50.40

*Based on estimates from the U. S. Agriculture Department as of late 1970. Costs given are for individuals in families of four. For one person, add 20 per cent; for a two-person family, 10 per cent; three-person, 5 per cent. For families larger than four, adjust by subtracting 5 per cent for five-person family and 10 per cent for six or more.

**Total adjusted for size of family.

COMPARATIVE PROTEIN COSTS

	Typical Price per Lb.	Grams Protein per Lb.*	Cost of 100 Gms. Protein
Beans with pork	18¢	27.7	65¢
Perch fillets, frozen	59	87.5	67
Beef liver	57	90.3	63
Broilers, oven-ready	39	57.4	68
Cheddar cheese	91	113.4	80
American processed cheese	89	105.2	85
Eggs	69 (doz.)	78.3(doz.)	88
Salmon, pink, canned	83	93.0	89
Cottage cheese, creamed	55	61.7	89
Tuna, chunk, canned	99	109.8	90
Turkey, oven-ready	59	65.9	90
Hamburger, regular	74	81.2	91
Halibut steaks	94	94.8	99
Beef chuck, with bone	74	71.6	$1.03
Fishsticks, breaded, frozen	80	76.0	$1.05
Flounder fillets, frozen	83	75.8	$1.09
Cod fillets	89	79.8	$1.12
Liverwurst, unsliced	84	73.5	$1.14
Frankfurters, regular	75	64.4	$1.16
Chili con carne, with beans, canned	40	34.0	$1.18
Ham, cured, with bone	82	68.3	$1.20
Luncheon meat, canned	86	68.0	$1.27
Bologna, unsliced	79	60.3	$1.31
Pork loin	80	61.1	$1.31
Frankfurters, all meat	79	59.4	$1.33
Corned beef hash, canned	54	39.9	$1.35
Liverwurst, sliced	$1.04	73.5	$1.42
Lamb, leg	98	67.7	$1.45
Salami, cooked	$1.18	79.4	$1.48
Beef tongue, smoked	89	57.7	$1.54
Dried beef, chipped	$2.68	155.6	$1.72
Bologna, sliced	$1.04	60.3	$1.73
Round steak, with bone	$1.59	88.5	$1.80
Boiled ham	$1.89	103.5	$1.83
Lamb, shoulder chops	$1.12	58.9	$1.90
Sirloin steak	$1.37	71.1	$1.93

	Typical Price per Lb.	Grams Protein per Lb.*	Cost of 100 Gms. Protein
Bacon, sliced	94¢	38.1	$2.4
Veal, rib chops	$1.64	65.7	$2.5

*As purchased–uncooked.

COSTS PER SERVING*

Item	Average Portion	Cost per Lb.	Cost per Serving
Cheese, mild cheddar	2 oz.	91¢	11¢
Breast of lamb	1/2-3/4 lb.	26	13-20
Beef liver	1/4 lb.	57	14
Smoked ham	1/4-1/2 lb.	63	16-31
Eggs	3	69(doz.)	17
Hamburger, regular	1/4-1/3 lb.	74	19-25
Frankfurters	1/4-1/3 lb.	79	20-26
Broilers, oven-ready	1/2-3/4 lb.	39	20-29
Beef tongue, smoked	1/4 lb.	89	22
Pork loin	1/3 lb.	80	26
Flounder fillets	1/3 lb.	83	28
Breast of veal	1/2 lb.	59	30
Cod fillets	1/3 lb.	89	30
Turkey	1/2-3/4 lb.	59	30-45
Lamb, shoulder	1/3-1/2 lb.	89	30-45
Lamb, leg	1/3-2/3 lb.	98	33-65
Haddock fillets	1/3 lb.	$1.02	34
Beef chuck, with bone	1/2 lb.	74	37
Lamb, shoulder chops	1/3-1/2 lb.	$1.12	37-56
Round steak	1/4 lb.	$1.59	40
Sirloin steak	3/8-3/4 lb.	$1.37	51¢-$1.03
Rib roast	1/2-3/4 lb.	$1.09	55-82

*The prices are as of 1970. "Servings" listed are those considered "nutritionally adequate"–usually, a quarter pound of lean meat or a half-pound with bone and fat. As prices change, relative costs, of course, will change too.

YIELD OF COOKED MEAT PER POUND OF RAW MEAT

Meat as purchased	Description	Approx. Yield per Lb. of Raw Meat
Chops or steaks for broiling or frying:		
With bone and relatively large amount of fat, such as: pork or lamb chops, beef rib, sirloin, or porterhouse steaks	With bone and fat	10-12 oz.
	Without bone, with fat	7-10
	Lean only	5-7
Without bone and with very little fat, such as: round of beef, veal steaks	Lean and fat	12-13
	Lean only	9-12
Ground meat for broiling or frying, market type, such as: hamburger, lamb or pork patties	Patties	9-13

Roasts for oven cooking:

With bone and relatively large amount of fat, such as: beef rib, loin, or chuck; lamb shoulder, leg; pork, fresh or cured

With bone and fat	10-12
Without bone, with fat	8-10
Lean only	6-9

Without bone

Lean and fat	10-12
Lean only	7-10

Cuts for potroasting, simmering, braising, stewing:

With bone and relatively large amount of fat, such as: beef chuck, pork shoulder

With bone and fat	10-11
Without bone, with fat	8-9
Lean only	6-8

Without bone and with relatively small amount of fat, such as: trimmed beef, veal

Lean, with small amount of adhering fat	9-11

Adapted from *Home and Garden Bulletin No. 72*, U. S. Agriculture Department.

HOW TO ESTIMATE COST
PER SERVING OF MEAT AND POULTRY*

Retail Cut	Servings per Lb.	29	39	49	59	69	79	89	99	109	119	129	139
		If price per pound is:											
		Cost per serving is:											
Beef:													
Sirloin steak	2-1/2	12	16	20	24	28	32	36	40	44	48	52	56
Porterhouse, T-bone, rib steak	2	15	20	25	30	35	40	45	50	55	60	65	70
Round steak	3-1/2	8	11	14	17	20	23	25	28	31	34	37	40
Chuck roast, bone-in	2	15	20	25	30	35	40	45	50	55	60	65	70
Rib roast, bone-in	2	15	20	25	30	35	40	45	50	55	60	65	70
Rump, sirloin roast	3	10	13	16	20	23	26	30	33	36	40	43	46
Ground beef	4	7	10	12	15	17	20	22	25	27	30	32	35
Short ribs	2	15	20	25	30	35	40	45	50	55	60	65	70
Heart, liver, kidney	5	6	8	10	12	14	16	18	20	22	24	26	28
Frankfurters	4	7	10	12	15	17	20	22	25	27	30	32	35
Stew meat, boneless	5	6	8	10	12	14	16	18	20	22	24	26	28
Lamb:													
Loin, rib, shoulder chops	3	10	13	16	20	23	26	30	33	36	40	43	46
Breast, shank	2	15	20	25	30	35	40	45	50	55	60	65	70
Shoulder roast	2-1/2	12	16	20	24	28	32	36	40	44	48	52	56
Leg of lamb	3	10	13	16	20	23	26	30	33	36	40	43	46
Pork—fresh:													
Center or rib chops	4	7	10	12	15	17	20	22	25	27	30	32	35
Loin or rib roast	2-1/2	12	16	20	24	28	32	36	40	44	48	52	56
Boston butt, bone-in	3	10	13	16	20	23	26	30	33	36	40	43	46
Spare ribs	1-1/3	22	29	37	44	52	59	67	74	82	89	97	104
Pork—cured:													
Picnic, bone-in	2	15	20	25	30	35	40	45	50	55	60	65	70
Ham, fully cooked:													
bone-in	3-1/2	8	11	14	17	20	23	25	28	31	34	37	40
boneless and canned	5	6	8	10	12	14	16	18	20	22	24	26	28
shankless	4-1/4	7	9	12	14	16	19	21	23	26	28	30	33
center slice	5	6	8	10	12	14	16	18	20	22	24	26	28
Poultry:													
Broiler, read-to-cook	1-1/3	22	29	37	44	52	59	67	74	82	89	97	104
legs, thighs,	3	10	13	16	20	23	26	30	33	36	40	43	46
breasts	4	7	10	12	15	17	20	22	25	27	30	32	35
Turkey, ready-to-cook, under 12 lbs.	1	29	39	49	59	69	79	89	99	109	119	129	139

*Adapted from *Food for Us All*, U. S. Agriculture Department, 1969.

15

PRICE JUGGLERS AND GENUINE SPECIALS

Planning meals around supermarket specials can be an important aid in restraining your food bills. In fact, often when food prices are high, stores tend to offer more specials to stimulate sales. Or when retail prices lag behind declines in farm prices, retailers often tend to offer specials rather than make more widespread reductions.

For example, if hog marketings increase in response to higher quotations, retailers may be reluctant to decrease prices generally, but may offer temporary specials on several pork cuts.

Thus, you almost have to shop the specials to beat the merchandising men at their own favorite game of juggling prices.

How much can you trust advertised specials? All the evidence is that you can make savings, but need to be alert to certain practices or omissions.

Stefan Josenhans checked advertised sales at three leading chain supermarkets in the New York metropolitan area for two weeks. On thirty-four specials, he found reductions from regular prices ranged from as little as 5 percent to as much as 37 percent.

But the fact of life which consumers need to know is that some specials are on staple, useful items, but others involve the more expensive brands or versions. These may not be as good value as the store's own brands or other national brands, even at the reduced prices.

The most useful specials are those on meats, canned and fresh produce and on stores' own brands of dry groceries. Already priced lower than the national brands, private brands on sale represent genuine opportunities to anticipate needs by buying in bulk quantities.

Of the thirty-four sale items, seventeen were on staple foods and private brands, including bacon, turkey roast, canned fruit juices, canned vegetables and fruits, paper goods and so on. The others featured such items as a national brand of frozen orange juice which did not meet the value of the private brands, even at its temporarily reduced price, and such specialties as whipped cream cheese, expensive brands of cake mixes and luxury canned soups, spaghetti sauces, chopped mushrooms, jumbo olives and a special pet food.

A detailed study in Manhattan, Kansas, by students of Dr. Richard Morse, head of the Family Economics Department at Kansas State University, found that about half the advertised specials were genuine.

The students checked prices in ten stores, including four chain supermarkets. They checked the advertised specials and noted their availability, and then came back two weeks and four weeks later to check the current prices of the same items.

The price checkers found that genuine specials in various stores ranged from one-fourth to nine out of ten of the items advertised, with an overall average of about half. Over half of the "specials" of the national chain supermarkets were the same price when checked two and four weeks later.

In contrast, our own price-checking found that ten of the thirty-four advertised specials were still the same price, or still "on sale" ten days later. This raises the question of whether they were actual specials or merely regular prices. Either way, these particular items were relatively good values.

The Kansas checkers found that "specials" of independent stores were more likely to be genuine. Two-thirds or more were featured at prices lower than prices two and four weeks later.

What about the availability of "specials"? Consumers often find they sometimes are not available when they get to the stores. One retired man reports that he went to a chain supermarket that had advertised a special on broilers. He found none. The manager explained that the trailer had not arrived yet. He went to another store but saw none of the broilers on the counter that it had advertised. He determinedly went right into the back room. The "sale" chickens were there all right—piled in a cart.

Many people, of course, who do not find "sale" items at the meat counter simply buy the "regular-price" items. Some of the more determined ones insist on getting the advertised special.

For that reason, some supermarkets now offer "rain checks." In fact, some of the more alert local weights and measures departments insist that they do. This is some help, but requires a return shopping trip, and is no substitute for honest advertising to start with, and careful checking by both the newspapers who publish the ads and weights and measures departments.

The Kansas students did find that 96 percent of the advertised items were available in the eight stores they checked. But other experiences indicate that the problem of availability most often occurs in the most important sale item—meats and poultry.

You also have to watch to make sure the items are actually marked with the "special" price. The Kansas students found some stores marked all the items with the special price, but others marked as few as one out of four. On the average, seven out of ten "sale" items were marked with the special price. If not, the check-out clerk may tend to charge the regular price.

In Josenhans' experience, absence of a marked sale price may be an oversight or the manager may have underestimated demand. There is a tendency to avoid marking down too many items to save rubbing out and remarking stock later. The proper procedure is for the checkers to have a list of the sale items and to charge only the advertised prices. The checkers are supposed at least to recognize the sale items, although part-time checkers who work on Saturdays may not be as aware of them.

The Kansas students also found indications that some stores advertised fictitiously high "regular" prices. The prices two and four weeks after the "sale" were lower than the previously quoted "regular" price.

A survey by the Federal Trade Commission in Washington, D.C., and San Francisco found that 11 percent of the advertised items in two cities were unavailable and that only 8 of the 137 stores operated by ten leading chains had every advertised item available.[15]

Significantly, the FTC also found that considerably more sale items were unavailable in low-income area stores than in higher-income areas.

Meat and poultry are the most important items to you. They also are the foods most often sale-priced, and so the key to planning your meals and even to which markets to use. Note the chart of seasonal variations in food prices in this chapter. Meats, in general, are relatively low in the spring, rise during the summer to a peak in September and then gradually decline during the winter.

The average variation in meat prices between highest and low months is only 4 percent. But the savings on meat specials are much more likely to range from 22 to 37 percent in our experience. One week in November, 1970, in the New York metropolitan area, turkey prices ranged from 59-69 cents a pound, but you could find specials as low as 45 cents. (You also could pay as much as 79 cents.) Or you could pay as little as 95 cents for round roast, when the usual range was $1.39 to $1.59.

The meat items most often on sale are chuck steak and broilers. You could pay anywhere from 29 to 53 cents for broilers in late 1970.

When pork is in heavy supply, especially in the spring, some cuts are used as really low-priced leaders. For example, one week in 1970 when meat prices generally were at high levels, the usual price for loin roast rib end was 69 cents. But there were many sales at 39 to 49 cents.

Sometimes consumers feel that meat specials are no better values because, it is said, specials are not trimmed as well or meat is of lower quality. This may have been true more in years past than now, when consumers have become increasingly conscious and articulate about heavy fat or even added fat. Additional confirmation was provided by a Consumers Union survey published in August, 1970. The survey found that specials did offer savings, whether or not the supermarkets trimmed less than usual from specials, and the quality of sale-priced beef was the same.

But there are differences in trimming practices among stores.

Fruits and vegetables are another leading area for specials with sharp differences in prices, as stores feature not only seasonal items but staples. Prices of specific produce items may vary as much as 50 percent among supermarkets in the same shopping area. Sale prices on canned fruits and vegetables are especially low in September, when stores clear the old pack in preparation for the new harvest.

One of the most persistent complaints is that stores sometimes do not pass on to consumers the "cents off" or other cash discounts offered by manufacturers from time to time.

Often the stores do not pass on the discounts, a survey by Thomas Jurkiewicz, a student of Dr. Stewart at Geneva College, found. Of the five stores Jurkiewicz studied, those advertising lower prices and "greater savings for your dollar" were those least likely to give the discount. One store simply tended to ignore the discounts.

A frequent practice was to raise the price to offset the discount, and then reduce the item back down to its regular price. One store would even put a new sticker over the old sticker, but with the same price.

Sometimes stores would give only part discounts. On "10-cents off" offers on detergents, the regular price was reduced only 7 cents in several instances.

Store practices varied. Two of the five stores, one a leading low-price chain and the other a higher-priced small store, did try to pass on the discounts.

One wholesaler's salesman told Jurkiewicz that he spends "over half his time" going back to stores and marking prices down to where they should be. It seems that after he leaves the store, the prices seem to get raised a little, as indicated by letters sent in by angry consumers.

Without any serious government intervention, Jurkiewicz's experience has led him to feel that only the consumer can put a stop to this deceit. First and foremost, he advised, call the "mismarked" item to the attention of the store management. He found that when he pointed out the discrepancies, managers did tend to reduce the prices.

You also can write to the president of the large chains and to the manufacturers to put pressure on the managers to reduce prices, he suggested.

In Washington, David Angevine even found one leading brand of expensive coffee imitating a "cents off" special. The label featured the figures "15" in large type. But underneath, in smaller type, was the word "points." The buyer would get fifteen points toward bonus gifts, or 2 ¼ cents in cash.

Under the Truth-in-Packaging law, the Food and Drug Administration is empowered to regulate "cents off" labeling on foods and cosmetics (the FTC on other items). In late 1970, as this is written, a pending regulation would require that such offers be made only if the product's retail selling price has been established and is reduced by at least the amount represented on the "cents off" label. This requirement would rule out some of the many incredible "cents off" offers on brand-new products or products being market-tested. Moreover, the offer could not last more than a month; coupons would have to be redeemable at the point of sale; packagers who label products "economy size" would have to demonstrate actual savings.[16]

Unfortunately, neither the FDA nor FTC regulations would provide controls on retailers who may neglect to pass on the "cents off" to consumers. The agencies were more or less hoping (vainly, in my opinion) that the manufacturers would police the retailers.

In any case, you may have observed that "cents off" coupons usually involve expensive new products such as synthetic dessert toppings and breakfast beverages, canned and packaged frostings and the more expensive brands of coffee. *U.S. Consumer* told about one coupon offer of 25 cents off on a 59-cent can of scalloped potatoes in "cream" sauce. The result was one generous serving of potatoes for 34 cents.

The purpose of specials, besides their useful role in moving seasonally abundant crops, is, of course, to bring traffic into the store to buy non-sale items. Supermarket displays obviously are arranged to encourage impulse buying; for example, products with more facings on a shalf sell more than those with narrow facings. Another practice, of which shoppers have complained, is advertising a special on, say, canned peaches, and then displaying large aisle-end stacks of peaches, but not those on sale. Stores also place their displays of coffee, a large volume item, to lead consumers past displays of impulse items.

Sometimes, too, you may arrive late on the last day of the sale and find the higher prices have been restored. Store personnel tend to start marking items back to the original price the afternoon before.

A frequent way of making it hard to compare prices or to know if a price has been reduced or increased, is the practice of juggling the number of units sold at a given price. The Agriculture Department has pointed out that switching an item from 18 cents each to two for 33 cents enables stores to feature a 3-cent reduction instead of 1½ cents. It works the other way, too. A change from two for 33 cents to 18 cents each can obscure a price increase.

Shoppers tend to submit to "twofer" and "threefer" pricing, even if they had not intended to buy several of that item. They even have been known to buy more of a 33-cent item if it is offered at three for 99 cents.

SEASONAL VARIATIONS IN FOOD PRICES*

Item	Jan.	Feb.	Mar.	Apr.	May	June	July	Aug.	Sept.	Oct.	Nov.	Dec.
Meats	99.8	99.5	98.8	98.5	98.0	98.2	100.3	101.7	102.4	101.8	100.6	100.0
Beef and veal	100.8	100.6	99.8	99.2	98.8	97.9	99.0	100.3	101.0	101.0	101.0	100.8
Round steak	100.3	100.6	99.5	99.2	99.0	98.1	99.6	100.5	100.3	101.6	100.9	100.6
Chuck roast	101.7	101.6	101.0	99.7	98.2	95.1	96.3	99.5	101.4	100.8	102.2	102.1
Hamburger	100.7	100.0	99.4	99.0	98.6	99.3	99.6	99.4	101.3	100.7	100.7	100.9
Pork	98.6	98.4	97.3	96.7	97.1	98.2	102.2	104.3	105.1	102.7	100.3	98.8
Pork chops	98.9	98.4	96.8	96.0	95.4	98.0	103.4	106.1	104.7	103.6	100.4	98.0
Ham, whole	101.1	100.4	99.4	98.8	97.4	98.4	99.5	101.1	101.1	100.5	100.5	101.3
Bacon	97.1	97.7	96.9	96.3	97.4	98.1	102.6	106.0	106.7	103.0	99.7	98.1
Other meats	99.9	99.8	99.6	99.6	99.8	100.0	99.8	100.1	100.7	100.5	100.3	100.0
Frankfurters	99.7	99.6	99.7	99.5	99.3	99.8	99.7	100.0	101.2	100.8	100.7	100.1
Chicken, frying	99.9	101.3	101.3	100.1	98.3	100.8	101.2	99.6	100.4	99.1	99.6	98.4
Fish	100.4	100.6	100.0	100.1	100.1	99.9	99.8	99.7	99.5	99.6	100.0	100.0
Fresh or frozen	100.4	100.6	100.0	100.2	100.2	99.6	99.8	99.8	99.8	99.6	99.9	99.9
Fresh milk, grocery	100.9	100.4	100.0	99.2	98.6	98.1	99.1	100.1	100.5	101.0	101.1	101.0
Eggs	103.9	102.5	97.4	96.4	90.5	88.3	92.4	97.4	109.7	110.4	106.5	105.0

Fresh fruits and vegetables												
	96.4	98.5	99.9	102.7	105.2	108.0	110.8	101.1	94.8	93.5	93.9	95.7
Apples	96.7	91.2	94.5	101.1	108.9	121.1	129.5	125.8	95.2	81.5	79.8	84.3
Bananas	96.4	101.3	100.3	100.1	99.9	100.8	99.6	100.6	101.0	103.1	99.0	98.2
Oranges	91.9	93.6	95.4	99.4	98.3	98.1	100.8	103.1	107.2	108.3	105.8	98.2
Grapefruit	86.9	89.1	88.1	89.8	95.2	106.9	113.2	116.4	116.7	117.0	93.2	87.3
Potatoes	93.5	94.8	95.0	97.6	103.8	115.3	123.1	105.9	95.8	92.6	91.5	91.9
Onions	95.2	96.9	96.8	102.4	103.8	109.0	112.6	109.2	95.4	92.5	91.4	94.2
Cabbage	110.7	113.1	112.2	107.0	110.0	109.5	98.8	89.4	86.4	87.4	84.9	90.7
Carrots	102.9	98.4	95.1	93.7	95.8	104.4	106.3	105.0	100.1	98.0	99.0	101.5
Celery	102.5	101.7	105.1	100.4	102.3	100.4	110.7	97.0	92.5	95.0	96.1	96.5
Lettuce	103.5	109.1	102.7	96.6	98.5	100.8	91.1	91.8	98.5	99.7	107.9	99.6
Tomatoes	114.9	106.0	112.6	116.4	116.8	105.2	110.1	73.3	68.3	74.1	90.2	111.3
Grapes	—	—	—	—	—	—	130.4	98.8	83.7	91.0	97.8	—
Strawberries	—	—	—	113.2	96.1	88.1	—	—	—	—	—	—
Watermelon	—	—	—	—	—	121.9	94.8	80.5	—	—	—	—
Frozen orange juice	102.9	101.4	100.9	100.7	98.5	97.8	98.4	98.8	98.8	99.2	100.7	102.1

*These indexes are based on annual average equal to 100, and are adapted from U. S. Bureau of Labor Statistics data.

16

WHERE STORES' OWN BRANDS
SAVE YOU MOST MONEY

Stores' own brands of packaged and canned foods cost 10 to 22 percent less than nationally advertised brands.

Savings on household cleaners and paper products are even larger, averaging 33 and 25 percent respectively on some widely used products.

These are several of the findings in a survey of private brands vs. national brands. The survey compared prices on identical or closely similar grades in one national chain, two regional chains and three local chains in two large cities and three smaller cities.

In all, Josenhans, who made the survey for this book, checked forty-five different items.

This and other surveys we have made have found some revealing differences in the cost per ounce for basically the same foods. In the case of peas, for example, there was a progression from a little over a penny an ounce, for stores' own brands of mixed-sized peas in a large can, to 2 ½ ounces for June peas in a small-sized nationally advertised brand.

Similarly, a small individual box of dry cereal in a nationally advertised brand costs more than twice as much per serving as a large box of private-brand cornflakes.

The largest price differences in individual items were 41 percent on margarine, 36 percent on frozen orange juice concentrate, 22 percent on white bread, 48 percent on puffed rice, 26 percent on cooked salami, 24 percent on salad dressing and 22 percent on nonfat dry milk.

In paper and cleaning products, the largest differences were on tissues, 39 percent, dishwashing detergent, 36 percent, liquid floor wax, 49 percent and plastic wrap, 39 percent.

In general, price differences were smallest, although still significant, on canned fruits and vegetables, ranging from only 5 percent on sliced peaches to as much as 22 percent on whole-kernel corn, and averaging 14 percent. Largest savings by categories were on frozen foods, particularly because of the big difference in costs of frozen orange juice. In coffee, the price difference was large for instant, small for ground.

A comparison we made in 1968 of private vs. national brands covering other items found especially large price differences in peanut butter (38 percent in smaller sizes), egg noodles (34 percent in small sizes, 28 percent in large), graham crackers (38 percent) and canned spinach (30 percent).

The dramatic differences between private and national-brand cleaning products shows how overpriced the heavily advertised detergents and specialty products really are. The 1968 survey also found such examples as Co-op Low-Sudsing Detergent selling for almost half the price of the leading national brand of that type. The small can of a famous brand of spray furniture wax costs 2 ½ times as much as the large can of a leading chain store's own brand. There were differences of 42 to 50 percent in prices of private and national-brand spray-can starches.

But not all private brands offer the same savings. Private-brand prices vary too. For example, one store's own brand of nonfat milk powder may save as much as 30 percent over a national brand. But another store's may save only 10 percent. One supermarket's own-brand bread may be as little as 20 cents a pound loaf; another's, 27. For instant coffee, private-brand prices ranged surprisingly—from 75 cents to $1.09 for 6-ounce jars.

Revealingly, we found almost all private brands cheaper, and significantly cheaper at two non-stamp chain stores than at two stamp-giving stores. On a list of twenty-one private-brand grocery items (no meat or fresh produce) the total cost at the two stamp-giving markets was $8.03 and $7.55, compared with $6.80

at the leading non-stamp store in the neighborhood. This is a difference of $1.23, or 18 percent.

But the stamp stores were closer to the prices of the non-stamp stores on national brands—in the case of the three neighboring stores, $9.50, $9.23 and $8.86. This was a difference of 64 cents, or 7 percent.

Evidently, the stamp-giving stores are competing to a greater degree on national brands, but taking additional margin on their own brands, which are less identifiable and harder to compare for value. In any case the higher costs, at least among the stores we compared, are more necessitated by the additional 2 percent or 2 cents on a dollar that stores pay for the trading stamps they give you.

Thus you do have to determine the comparative costs of the private brands of different retailers in your own area. Another study, in 1966, reported by Don Lefever, grocery supervisor for District of Columbia area co-ops, found the same list of private brands cost $10.78, $11.57, $12.17 and $12.18 at four different stores, compared with $13.71 for the same list in national brands.

How good are private brands? They usually are good quality, packed for the retailers according to specifications, and sometimes processed in retailers' own factories. Often, in fact, the private brands are similar to or even the same as the national brands.

For example, of four brands of canned small early peas we checked, ranging in price from 25 to 33 cents for cans marked 17 ounces, all had within 10¾ and 11¼ ounces of solid content. The cheapest, a private brand, was exactly in the middle, with 11 ounces of actual peas. They were similar in tenderness and size, with the lowest-priced brand again ranking in the middle in size and tenderness, one national brand ranking below it and the other two—a private brand at 27 cents and a national brand at 33 cents—ranking on top with smaller peas.

In Chapter 3 it also was noted that a private-brand frozen dinner which cost 45 cents actually had an ounce more beef than the leading national brand. (If you have ever eaten one of these heat-and-serve dinners, you know that an ounce is important.)

This similar or even identical quality has even been the subject of court cases. I have reported before that Borden's was told by the Federal Trade Commission to stop charging retailers more for canned milk of "like grade and quality" sold under its own name than they charged for milk sold under retailers' labéls. [17] In the similar "Florida Beverage" case, the courts also found that the private-label liquors and national-advertised liquors sold by this distributor were of like grade and quality. The only difference was the different labels, Francis Mayer of the Federal Trade Commission has pointed out.

SAVINGS ON PRIVATE BRANDS

Fruits and Vegetables

Sliced peaches, 29 oz.	5.0%
Bartlett pears, 16 oz.	20.4
Applesauce, 25-oz. jar	9.7
Early small peas, 16 oz.	14.0
Whole kernel corn, 16 oz.	22.0
	Avg: 14.2%

Drinks and Juices

Fruit drinks, 46 oz.	19.6%
Tomato juice, 46 oz.	18.0
	Avg: 18.8%

Coffee

Ground, 1 lb.	8.4%
Instant, 6 oz.	19.6
	Avg: 14.0%

Frozen Foods

Orange juice concentrate, 6 oz.	35.9%
Peas, 10 oz.	16.8
Mixed vegetables, 10 oz.	19.3
Corn, 10 oz.	14.7
Pot pies, 8 oz.	24.4
	Avg: 22.2%

Dairy

Skim milk, ½ gal.	6.4%
Cottage cheese, lb.	12.6
Soft margarine, lb.	21.2
Stick margarine, lb.	40.8
American cheese, 12 oz. (wrapped slices)	7.2
Swiss cheese, 8 oz.	11.7
	Avg: 16.6%

Meats

Bacon	33.9%
Bologna	15.6
Cooked salami	25.5
Franks (all types)	3.4
	Avg: 19.6%

Canned Meats and Fish

Corned beef hash, 16 oz.*	7.2%
Luncheon meat, 12 oz.	8.5
Tuna, 7 oz. (solid white)	15.8
	Avg: 10.5%

Paper Products

Tissues, 200's	39.2%
Aluminum foil, 25 ft.	18.0
Plastic wrap	29.4
	Avg: 25.5%

Cleaning Products

Dishwashing detergent, 22 oz.	36.6%
Powdered cleanser, 14 oz.	33.3
Liquid bleach, ½ gal.	14.3
Liquid floor wax, 27 oz.*	49.0
	Avg: 33.4%

Bread and Cereal

White bread, 1 lb.	22.4%
Round crackers, 12 oz.*	19.6
Corn flakes, 12 oz.	10.6
Puffed rice, 6 oz.	47.8
Corn flakes, 18 oz.	9.5
	Avg: 22.0%

Miscellaneous Groceries

Nonfat dry milk, 8 qt.	21.8%
Spaghetti, lb.	18.5
Salad dressing, 8 oz. (liquid)	23.8
Peanut butter, 12 oz.	10.0
Pancake syrup, 24 oz.	14.0
Corn oil, 48 oz.	8.5
	Avg: 16.1%

*Closest sizes adjusted for price averaging.

CHAPTER

17

A GRADE BY ANY OTHER
NAME IS JUST THE SAME

Buying by grade is one of the most useful techniques available to
you for keeping down family food bills. There are instances in
which you save almost half the cost of an item by buying
according to grade rather than brand name. As one of many
examples, we found seven different brands of frozen orange juice
concentrate all labeled "U.S. Grade A." They were priced at 14,
15, 16 (several) and 25 cents—a difference of 80 percent from
lowest to highest. You could have bought any of them with
assurance that you were getting the same high quality. In fact,
most of the private brands are packed by the same Florida
packing plant under different labels.

The U.S. grade marks on meat, poultry, eggs, cheese, canned
fruits and vegetables and other foods assure you that you get
specific, uniform quality, no matter what the price or brand
name or where you buy. For example, beef marked "U.S.
Choice" has been graded by government experts and meets the
standard for this quality, no matter who sells it.

Many retailers require that wholesalers sell to them on the
basis of government grades to make sure that they—the
retailers—get the quality they pay for. Unfortunately, showing
the grade on the consumer package is voluntary, not mandatory.
Thus, some of the same retailers do not show the government grade when they, in turn, sell to us. Some merely use

meaningless brand names on their own versions or grade designations on meats and other food products. The government's own standards names are sometimes fanciful enough. For example, the designation "Large" on shrimp really is for the medium size. Larger than "Large" are "Extra Large," "Jumbo," "Extra Jumbo," "Colossal" and "Extra Colossal."

If grading were required by law right down to the retail counter, your buying problems would be simplified. Some manufacturers and stores do state in their ads and on packages what the grade is. As for the others, you have every right to ask the meat department manager just what grade of meat he is selling, and to show you the U.S. grade mark.

This already has happened in the case of broilers, turkeys and other poultry, to the benefit of both consumers and the poultry industry. Since broilers have become a modern mainstay of family dinners because of their low modern prices and the high prices of red meat, the fact that many processors now grade-label broilers enables you to buy any broiler marked U.S. Grade A, whether it is 29 or 49 cents a pound.

In our price surveys for this book, we also found turkeys priced all the way from 49 to 79 cents a pound, with the same U.S. Grade A label. Thus, we were sure, and visual inspection confirmed, that the turkeys at the lower price met the specifications for high quality: broad-breasted, fully-fleshed, with good appearance and conformation, and free from defects such as cuts and bruises.

Here is the technique of using to your advantage what grades are available:

—Understand, first of all, that the grade has nothing to do with food value. All grades, whether "Choice" or "Good" beef, Grade A or Grade B eggs, "Fancy" or "No. 1" apples, have the same food value. The higher grades merely have better appearance and more uniform size, and, in the case of meat, may be juicier, and sometimes—not always—more tender. In fact, sometimes, as in the case of meat, the lower grades usually have more protein and vitamin value.

Supermarket chains traditionally offer the lower grades cheap as a leader, and then have one or two higher-priced grades on which they make a bigger profit.

Not only do such grades help you select the best value,

without depending solely on advertised names, but grades also help you choose the right quality for the intended use. Usually the chief difference between the grades is appearance and uniform size of the pieces.

In canned string beans, for example, the Grade A are uniform in appearance and color, Grade B is almost as attractive in appearance and Grade C consists of short-cut beans of varying size, and possibly less tenderness. The most expensive grade is rarely worth buying. The Grade B is an all-purpose grade, which can be bought when appearance is important. But Grade C is the best buy when the cooking method is going to change the appearance, texture and even flavor, as in a stew.

Another example is canned tomatoes. The Grade A provides whole tomatoes of uniform shape, free from defects and with red color. Grade B provides large pieces and even some whole tomatoes with defects removed. Grade C tomatoes are smaller pieces, but perfectly satisfactory for stews and other cooking purposes, at almost half the price of some Grade A brands.

Usually in canned fruits and vegetables, a moderate-income family's best buy is Grade B, or if not government graded, the store's second grade. For example, in peaches, for a difference of ten cents or more a can, you will find that Grade C has irregular pieces, while the Grade A is uniform. But except for a heavier syrup (sugar and water) the difference in flavor is minor.

In general, the policy I have recommended for many years is to buy Grade A for the table and Grade B for the pot. In eggs, for example, the yolk of Grade B eggs is a little flatter and not as thick, and the flavor is a little less delicate than in the Grade A. You might want Grade A for boiling or frying, but Grade B is just as satisfactory for omelets, casseroles and other cooking and baking purposes.

In beef and veal, the official U.S. grades are U.S. Prime, Choice, Good and Standard. Good grade usually is the best buy in protein and vitamin value because not only is the price less than the Choice, but Good grade is comparatively lean. The Good has less fat (18 percent) than the costlier Choice grade, which is 25 percent fat and so is less juicy, but is relatively tender. Usually, the Good grade requires longer, moist cooking methods, as in braising or stewing.

You may not, however, be able to find the Good grade in all

stores. Many handle just one grade—usually Choice. Some who offer two grades may handle Choice and Prime, although Prime is not often sold in retail markets, but more usually goes to restaurants. Others, more often in moderate-income large-city neighborhoods, may offer a Choice and Good grade, but may call the Good grade by another name, such as Economy grade.

Because meat often does not carry the government grade label after the stores cut it up, you may get the Good grade anyway, thinking you are getting Choice and perhaps paying the price for Choice. Most people, when asked to identify different grades of beef, usually choose the Good or even Standard grade as the top quality. The lower grades look better to them because they have less fat.

Only beef, veal and lamb have government grades. Pork does not.

As noted, poultry often carries the U.S. grade; meats, sometimes; canned and frozen fruits, sometimes; fruit juice concentrates often do; fresh fruits and vegetables, infrequently. Eggs often may be graded and labeled according to your state marketing laws, which are not uniform and sometimes tend to favor eggs produced on local farms rather than those shipped in from other states.

To get maximum usefulness from whatever U.S. grade designations are available in stores in your area, you do need to know the marks used for various foods. Most are letter designations. There is some tendency to give high-sounding designations to even medium quality, sometimes at the sacrifice of uniformity in designation. For example, while for poultry the top grade is U.S. "A," for cheddar cheese "A" is the second grade, and the top grade is "AA." A number of the more widely used food grades are provided in the following chart.

GOVERNMENT FOOD GRADES*

Beef, veal, lamb	U. S. Prime, Choice, Good, Standard
Poultry	U. S. Grades A and B
Eggs	U. S. Grades AA, A and B (Also classified for size: extra large, large, medium, small)
Cheese	Federal grades for cheddar cheese are U. S. Grade AA or A, but these may not often appear on retail packages. There are no grades for processed cheeses, cheese "foods" and cottage cheese, but these may carry a USDA "quality approved" shield if manufactured in an approved plant and the cheese meets federal standards of identity.
Butter	U. S. Grades AA, A and B
Canned, frozen, dried fruits, vegetables	U. S. Grade A or U. S. Fancy; U. S. Grade B or U. S. Choice; U. S. Extra Standard; U. S. Grade C or U. S. Standard
Rice, lentils, dry beans, dry peas	U. S. No. 1 or 2
Nonfat dry milk	U. S. Extra Grade (single quality grade)
Apples	U. S. Extra Fancy, Fancy, No. 1, Utility
Other fresh fruit, vegetables	Wholesale grades such as U. S. No. 1, 2, etc., may carry through to retail markets. Consumer grades, U. S. Grade A, B, etc., are used on a few products.

*Official USDA grades are shown in a shield and say "U. S."; for example, "U. S. Grade A." Unofficial grades such as simply "Grade A" or "Fancy" may be merely the packer's own designation, or in some cases, a state grade.

18

LARGER SIZES SAVE
18 PERCENT AND MORE

You do save by buying larger sizes. On the average, you save 18 percent by buying the large or medium size of a food product instead of the small, and 10 percent more by buying the extra-large, our surveys find.

In fact, the potential savings on some products are 50 percent and more. The true cost of foods and cleaning products in some of the small packages can surprise you if you figure out the actual cost per pound. The most expensive example, of the fifty-one items checked, is dry cereal packed in individual servings. These ten-package assortments have a true cost of approximately 80 cents a pound, compared with about 40 cents a pound for a standard dry cereal such as cornflakes in an 8-ounce box.

The savings on large sizes of household cleaners is smaller. In a few instances, the extra-large containers even cost as much as the medium-sized containers. This was found to be true in several brands of floor wax, and some of the liquid and powder detergents.

In general, however, we have found that the large sizes of cleaning products save 15 percent over the small, and the extra-large save 13 percent over the large (or more precisely, medium size).

In both foods and cleaners, the highest relative prices for

small sizes are among some of the nationally advertised brands. These often appear to be priced out of proportion to a normal differential between a small and large package.

Anastasio points out stores are very competitive on the 303 sizes (16 ounces) and cut prices on them, but take a higher margin on the smaller sizes such as the 8-ounce cans. Unfortunately poorer families especially tend to buy the 8-ounce sizes.

There is less price disparity between the small and larger sizes of retailers' own brands—the so-called "private brands." For example, the small size of an advertised brand of beans costs 17 percent more than a retailer's own brand. But in the large sizes the cost difference drops to about 6 percent. In canned corn, the price difference among small sizes was found to be as much as 28 percent, but only 13 percent in larger sizes.

There are two money-saving points to glean from these facts:

—Even for small families, the small sizes do not pay. You could "waste" up to a third of some of the larger sizes and still save over the extra-high prices of small containers. The real money-saving trick, of course, is to buy the larger sizes and then plan meals to use the extra quantity in different ways. Home economists and food processors who tell people to avoid waste by buying "only what you need" are not giving realistic advice.

In buying meats and poultry, it costs less to buy the whole ham than either of the halves, the pork loin rather than the chops and the whole bird rather than any of the parts, as shown in Chapter 10.

Turkey is an interesting example. For Thanksgiving, 1970, you could buy a 17-pound turkey for 59 cents a pound (about $10 for the whole bird) or a 12-pound turkey at 69 cents (about $8.30).

The larger turkey yields more meat per pound—about 55 percent, compared with 50 percent for the smaller bird. So the savings would be even greater. The cost for a three-quarter pound serving (11-12 ounces) from the smaller bird would be 51 cents. About 10 ounces of the larger bird would yield the same amount of meat, at a cost of 37 cents. In all, you would get twenty-seven servings from the $10 turkey and fifteen from the $8 one. The additional servings cost you only 18 cents each. A small family could afford even to give part of the turkey away, or share it with a neighbor.

—If you must buy a small size, make sure to get the store's own brand to avoid a disproportionately high overcharge (in most cases).

While the biggest savings are on the medium sizes over the small, large families can make additional worthwhile savings on extra-large containers. These are not available on all brands, but are found more often on the private brands. These money-savers include such extra-large sizes as a 3-pound box of macaroni and spaghetti, a 3- or 4-pound jar of peanut butter, soap pads boxed 18 or more, 21-ounce sizes of pork and beans and a 4-pound box of nonfat dry milk.

If you take the trouble to compute the cost per ounce, you will make some illuminating discoveries. For example, you will be able to see that in some stores Mr. Clean costs 2.6 cents an ounce in the small size, 2.46 cents in the medium size and 2.48 cents in the large. Top Job costs 2.6 cents an ounce in the 15-ounce size, 2.32 cents in the 1-pint, 12-ounce size and 2.43 cents in the 1-quart, 8-ounce size.

Why do you sometimes find that larger sizes actually cost more per ounce than smaller ones? This is not because of price juggling by the manufacturer, but because sometimes retailers in an area will tend to compete on a certain popular size and "discount" or cut the more normal price. When I pointed out this example to Procter & Gamble, who make both Mr. Clean and Top Job, they reported that their cost-per-ounce prices to the stores at that time were: 40-ounce size, 2.005 cents per ounce; 28-ounce size, 2.036; 5-ounce size, 2.113.

So do compute. You really only have to do it once in a while, since prices do not change every day. You will discover some other revealing facts. For example, Pledge furniture wax in a 7-ounce can for 79 cents comes to $1.80 a pint (16 ounces). A private-brand spray wax is almost half the price.

Also note the soap pads, especially the 4-pad box which comes out to 3.4 cents a pad, compared with a little over 2 cents for some of the private brands in boxes of ten or more.

In other food and cleaning products too often you will find that the combination of buying (1) the private brand in the (2) simplest version and (3) largest size can reduce the cost approximately by half.

SOME ESPECIALLY LARGE SAVINGS

	Small Size, Cost per Lb.	Medium Size, Cost per Lb.	Per Cent Saving
Pork and beans	25¢	17¢	33%
Canned peas	32	25.6	20
Egg noodles	50	40	20
Peanut butter	67	50	25
Salad dressing	54	39	48
Soda crackers	57	35	39
Snack crackers	62	45	27

APPENDIX

STANDARDS FOR CANNED AND PROCESSED MEAT, POULTRY AND FISH PRODUCTS

To be labeled with a particular name—such as "All Beef Franks" or "Chicken Soup"—a federally inspected meat or poultry product must be approved by the U.S. Department of Agriculture as meeting specific product requirements. Administration of these standards is under the Consumer and Marketing Service of the USDA. Following are products for which percentages of meat, poultry or other ingredients have been established. (This list does not include all products for which requirements have been set, nor does it necessarily include all requirements for those products that are listed.)

MEAT PRODUCTS

(All percentages of meat are on the basis of fresh *uncooked* weight, unless otherwise indicated):

—BARBECUED MEATS: Weight of meat when barbecued cannot exceed 70% of the weight of the fresh uncooked meat.

—BARBECUE SAUCE WITH MEAT: At least 35% meat (cooked basis).

—BEANS WITH BACON IN SAUCE: At least 12% bacon.

—BEANS WITH FRANKFURTERS IN SAUCE: At least 20 franks.

—BEANS WITH HAM IN SAUCE; At least 12% ham (cooked basis).

—BEEF WITH BARBECUE SAUCE: At least 50% beef (cooked basis).

—BEEF WITH GRAVY: At least 50% beef (cooked basis). If labeled GRAVY WITH BEEF: At least 35% beef (cooked basis).

—BEEF SAUSAGE (raw): No more than 30% fat.

—BEEF STROGANOFF: At least 45% fresh uncooked beef or 30% cooked beef, and at least 10% sour cream.

—BREADED STEAKS, CHOPS, etc.: Breading cannot exceed 30% finished product weight.

—BREAKFAST SAUSAGE: No more than 50% fat.

—BURRITOS: At least 15% meat.

—CHILI CON CARNE: At least 40% meat.

—CHILI CON CARNE WITH BEANS: At least 25% meat.

—CHILI SAUCE WITH MEAT: At least 6% meat.

—CHOP SUEY (AMERICAN STYLE) WITH MACARONI AND MEAT: At least 25% meat.

—CHOP SUEY VEGETABLES WITH MEAT: At least 12% meat.

—CHOW MEIN VEGETABLES WITH MEAT: At least 12% meat.

—CONDENSED, CREAMED DRIED BEEF OR CHIPPED BEEF: At least 18% dried or chipped beef (figured on reconstituted total content).

—CORN DOG: Must meet standards for frankfurters and batter cannot exceed the weight of the frank.

—CORNED BEEF AND CABBAGE: At least 25% corned beef.

—DEVILED HAM: No more than 35% fat.

—EGG FOO YUNG WITH MEAT: At least 12% meat.

—ENCHILADA WITH MEAT: At least 15% meat.

—EGG ROLLS WITH MEAT: At least 10% meat.

—FRANKFURTERS, BOLOGNA, OTHER COOKED SAUSAGE: May contain meat and meat by-products; no more than 30% fat, 10% added water and 2% corn syrup; no more than 15% poultry unless its presence is reflected in product name; no more than 3.5% cereals and nonfat dry milk, with product name showing that they are added. If labeled ALL MEAT, only muscle tissue with natural amounts of fat; no by-products, cereal or binders. If labeled ALL BEEF, only meat of beef animals may be used.

—FRITTERS: At least 35% meat.

—FROZEN BREAKFASTS: At least 15% meat (cooked basis).

—FROZEN DINNERS: At least 25% meat or meat food products (cooked basis, figured on total meat minus appetizer, bread and dessert).

—HAM: Not permitted to weigh more after processing than the fresh ham weighs before curing and smoking. Hams containing up to 10% added water must be labeled as HAM—WATER ADDED. If added water exceeds 10%, must be labeled IMITATION HAM.

—HAMBURGER OR GROUND BEEF: No more than 30% fat.

—HAM AND CHEESE SPREAD: At least 25% ham (cooked basis).

—HAM CHOWDER: At least 10% ham (cooked basis).
—HAM CROQUETTES: At least 35% ham (cooked basis).
—HAM SPREAD: At least 50% ham.
—HASH: At least 35% meat (cooked basis).
—LASAGNA WITH MEAT AND SAUCE: At least 12% meat.
—LIMA BEANS WITH HAM OR BACON IN SAUCE: At least 12% ham or cooked bacon.
—LIVER SAUSAGE, LIVER LOAF, LIVER PASTE, LIVER CHEESE, LIVER PUDDING, LIVER SPREAD AND SIMILAR LIVER PRODUCTS: At least 30% liver.
—MACARONI AND CHEESE WITH HAM: At least 12% ham (cooked basis).
—MACARONI AND BEEF IN TOMATO SAUCE: At least 12% beef.
—MEAT CASSEROLES: At least 25% fresh uncooked meat or 18% cooked meat.
—MEAT PIES: At least 25% meat.
—MEAT RAVIOLI: At least 10% meat in ravioli, minus the sauce.
—MEAT TACOS: At least 15% meat.
—MEAT TURNOVERS: At least 25% meat.
—OMELET WITH BACON: At least 12% bacon (cooked basis).
—OMELET WITH HAM: At least 18% ham (cooked basis).
—PEPPER STEAKS: At least 30% beef (cooked basis).
—PIZZA WITH MEAT: At least 15% meat.
—PIZZA WITH SAUSAGE: At least 12% sausage (cooked basis) or 10% dry sausage, such as pepperoni.
—PORK SAUSAGE: Not more than 50% fat.
—PORK WITH BARBECUE SAUCE: At least 50% pork (cooked basis).
—SAUERKRAUT WITH WIENERS AND JUICE: At least 20% wieners.
—SCALLOPED POTATOES AND HAM: At least 20% ham (cooked basis).
—SCALLOPINE: At least 35% meat (cooked basis).
—SCRAPPLE: At least 40% meat and/or meat by-products.
—SPAGHETTI SAUCE WITH MEAT: At least 6% meat.
—SPAGHETTI SAUCE AND MEAT BALLS: At least 35% meat balls (cooked basis).
—SPAGHETTI WITH MEAT AND SAUCE: At least 12% meat.

—SPAGHETTI WITH MEAT BALLS AND SAUCE: At least 12% meat.

—SPANISH RICE WITH BEEF OR HAM: At least 20% beef or ham (cooked basis).

—STEWS (BEEF, LAMB AND THE LIKE): At least 25% meat.

—SUKIYAKI: At least 30% meat.

—SWEET AND SOUR PORK OR BEEF: At least 25% fresh uncooked meat or 16% cooked meat, and at least 16% fruit.

—SWISS STEAK WITH GRAVY: At least 50% meat (cooked basis). If labeled GRAVY AND SWISS STEAK, at least 35% meat (cooked basis).

—TAMALES: At least 25% meat.

—TAMALES WITH SAUCE (OR WITH GRAVY): At least 20% meat.

—TONGUE SPREAD: At least 50% tongue.

—VEAL BIRDS: At least 60% meat and not more than 40% stuffing.

—VEAL FRICASSEE: At least 40% meat.

—VEAL PARMIGIANA: At least 40% breaded meat product in sauce. Breaded meat portion, at least 28% meat (cooked basis).

—VEAL STEAKS: Can be chopped, shaped, cubed, frozen. Beef can be added with product name shown as VEAL STEAKS, BEEF ADDED, CHOPPED, SHAPED AND CUBED. No more than 20% beef or must be labeled VEAL AND BEEF STEAK, CHOPPED, SHAPED AND CUBED. No more than 30% fat.

POULTRY PRODUCTS

(All percentages of poultry—chicken, turkey or other kinds—are on *cooked* deboned basis, unless otherwise indicated):

—BREADED POULTRY: No more than 30% breading.

—CANNED BONED POULTRY:

BONED, SOLID PACK: At least 95% poultry meat, skin and fat.

BONED: At least 90% poultry meat, skin and fat.

BONED, WITH BROTH: At least 80% poultry meat, skin and fat.

BONED, WITH SPECIFIED PERCENTAGE OF BROTH: At least 50% poultry meat skin and fat.

—CHICKEN CACCIATORE: At least 20% chicken meat, or 40% with bone.

—CHICKEN CROQUETTES: At least 25% chicken meat.

—CHOPPED POULTRY WITH BROTH (BABY FOOD): At least 43% poultry meat, with skin, fat and seasoning.

—CREAMED POULTRY: At least 20% poultry meat.

—POULTRY A LA KING: At least 20% poultry meat.

—POULTRY BARBECUE: At least 40% poultry meat.

—POULTRY BURGERS: 100% poultry meat, with skin and fat.

—POULTRY CHOP SUEY (SUCH AS CHICKEN CHOP SUEY): At least 4% poultry meat. If labeled CHOP SUEY WITH POULTRY, at least 2% poultry meat.

—POULTRY CHOW MEIN, WITHOUT NOODLES: At least 4% poultry meat.

—POULTRY DINNERS: At least 18% poultry meat.

—POULTRY FRICASSEE: At least 20% poultry meat.

—POULTRY FRICASSEE OF WINGS: At least 40% poultry meat (cooked basis, with bone).

—POULTRY HASH: At least 30% poultry meat.

—POULTRY NODDLES OR DUMPLINGS: At least 15% poultry meat, or 30% with bone. If labeled NOODLES OR DUMPLINGS WITH POULTRY, at least 6% poultry meat.

—POULTRY PIES: At least 14% poultry meat.

—POULTRY RAVIOLI: At least 2% poultry meat.

—POULTRY ROLLS: Binding agents limited to 3% in cooked roll.

—POULTRY SALAD: At least 25% poultry meat.

—POULTRY SOUP: At least 2% poultry meat.

—POULTRY STEW: At least 12% poultry meat.

—POULTRY TAMALES: At least 6% poultry meat.

—POULTRY TETRAZZINI: At least 15% poultry meat.

—POULTRY WITH GRAVY: At least 35% poultry meat. If labeled GRAVY WITH POULTRY, at least 15% poultry meat.

—SLICED POULTRY WITH GRAVY: At least 35% poultry.

STANDARDS OF IDENTITY

Complete standards of identity currently exist for two meat products. These standards require specific ingredients to be present as follows:

—CORNED BEEF HASH: Must contain at least 35% beef (cooked basis). Also must contain potatoes (either fresh, dehydrated, cooked dehydrated or a mixture of these types), curing agents and seasonings. May be made with certain optional ingredients such as onions, garlic, beef broth or beef fat. May not contain more than 15% fat nor more than 72% moisture.

—CHOPPED HAM: Must contain fresh, cured or smoked ham, along with certain specified kinds of curing agents and seasonings. May also contain certain optional ingredients in specified amounts, including finely chopped ham shank meat, dehydrated onions, dehydrated garlic, corn syrup, other chemical substances as permitted in the federal standard and not more than 3% water to dissolve the curing agents.

FROZEN FISH PRODUCTS

—FRIED FISH STICKS: At least 60% fish.
—FRIED BREADED FISH PORTIONS: At least 65% fish.
—RAW BREADED FISH PORTIONS: At least 75% fish.
—BREADED SHRIMP: At least 50% shrimp.
—LIGHTLY-BREADED SHRIMP: At least 65% shrimp.

USEFUL REFERENCES

The Co-Op Low Cost Cook Book. Berkeley: Consumers Cooperatives of Berkeley, 1969. (Address is 1414 University Ave., Berkeley, Calif.; paper cover, 95¢.)

Dyer, Ceil. *The Back to Cooking Cookbook.* Los Angeles: Price/Stern/Sloan, 1970. ($4.95)

Food and Drug Administration, Washington, D.C. 20204. *Read the Label.* (Tells what to look for on the labels of foods, drugs, cosmetics; single copies, free.)

   What Consumers Should Know about Food Standards. (Describes how standards are set; single copies, free.)

Gordon, Leland. *Weights and Measures and the Consumer.* Distributed by Consumers Union of U.S., Mt. Vernon, N.Y., 1970. (Thorough examination of practices; of special value to marketing students, teachers and officials; $3.)

Moolman, Valerie. *How to Buy Food.* New York: Cornerstone Library, 1970. (Concise, well-organized digest of information from government sources on shopping, quality guides, servings and care of foods; paper cover, $1.)

Office of Information, U.S. Department of Agriculture, Washington, D.C. 20250. *How to Buy Beef Roasts.* Home and Garden Bulletin No. 146. (Free.)

   Money Saving Dishes. Home and Garden Bulletin No. 43. (Free or, if no longer available, 30¢ from Superintendent of Documents.)

   . *Shopper's Guide to U.S. Grades of Food.* Home and Garden Bulletin No. 58. (Free.)

Stewart, Maxwell S. *Hunger in America.* Public Affairs pamphlet No. 457. (Available from Public Affairs Committee, 381 Park Avenue So., New York, N.Y. 10016; 25¢.)

Superintendent of Documents, Government Printing Office, Washington, D.C. 20402. *Family Fare.* (A daily food guide to kinds and amounts of foods to have each day; tips on meal planning; menu suggestions; 45¢.)

   . *Family Food Budgeting for Good Meals and Good Nutrition.* (Guides to budgeting at different cost levels with food plans; 15¢.)

. *Food for the Family with Young Children.* (Based on the food needs of a typical young couple with two pre-school children; provides suggestions on planning meals; also, tips for the proper diet for the expectant mother; 10¢.)

. *Food for Us All.* (1969 Yearbook of Agriculture; $3.50 or your Congressman still may be able to supply a free copy.)

. *How to Buy Canned and Frozen Vegetables.* (30¢)

. *How to Buy Fresh Fruits.* Home and Garden Bulletin No. 141. (15¢)

. *How to Buy Fresh Vegetables.* Home and Garden Bulletin No. 143. (15¢)

. *Nutritive Value of Foods.* Home and Garden Bulletin No. 72. (30¢)

NOTES

1. Economic Research Service, USDA, Bulletin ERS-446, October, 1970.
2. Reported by Cooperative News Service, Cooperative League of the U.S.A., May 19, 1970.
3. R.O. Herrmann and R.H. Warland in *Box Score on New Imitation Foods,* leaflet published by Cooperative Extension Service, Pennsylvania State University, University Park, Pa. 16802
4. Reported by R.S. Corken and P.B. Dwoskin in *Consumer Acceptance of A New Bacon Substitute,* ERS-454, Economic Research Service, USDA, October, 1970.
5. Quoted in *Supermarket News,* October 12, 1970.
6. From *Agricultural Markets in Change,* Agricultural Economic Report No. 95, 1966.
7. From *Composition of Foods,* Agriculture Handbook No. 8, U.S. Agriculture Department, revised Dec. 1963.
8. *Supermarket News,* Nov. 9, 1970.
9. *Canadian Consumer,* July/August, 1970.
10. A revealing report on such anticompetitive practices can be found in *Price Wars in City Milk Markets,* Agricultural Economic Report No. 100, 1966.
11. From the 1947-49 base period to autumn, 1970, the overall costs of food used at home rose 29 percent, while the price of white bread rose 35 percent. In contrast, Bureau of Labor Statistics data show that cookies went up 7 percent, whole wheat bread, 26 percent, and flour, 13. Even cornflakes, representative of the booming high-cost dry-cereal industry, went up just 30 percent.
12. *Christian Science Monitor,* March 11, 1970.
13. *Newsday,* Long Island, N.Y., October 30, 1970.
14. Marketing students and consumer-education teachers interested in this study can get it from the Superintendent of Documents, Washington, D.C., 20402; (*Consumers' Knowledge and Use of Government Grades for Selected Food Items,* USDA. Economic Research Service, Marketing Research Report No. 876.)
15. Economic Report on Food Chain Selling Practices in the District of Columbia and San Francisco, Bureau of Economics, Federal Trade Commission, Washington, D.C., July, 1969.
16. John Gomilla, the FDA official working on the proposed regulations, publicly lamented the fact that consumers were not aware of the proposed regulations on their behalf, and few had made comments during the three and a half months set aside for that purpose. In that period the FDA had received thirty-eight comments from industry representatives giving their views on the proposed rules, five from state officials—but only six from the entire consuming public. This appeared not to be apathy as much as sheer ignorance of what was going on. TV and newspapers did not report on this nonviolent happening, Gomilla observed.
17. *The Innocent Consumer vs. The Exploiters,* Trident Press, 1967.

INDEX

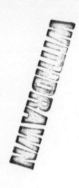